PRAISE FOR
The Patient-Centered Payoff

"The new era of healthcare reform ushers in new demands and higher expectations by patients—pressures pushing medical practices, large and small, to invoke a higher set of service standards in order to survive and thrive. Capko and Bisera deliver a precise roadmap for practices striving for success amidst an ever-changing landscape of rules, requests and requirements.

Learn how to analyze and respond to market forces. *The Patient-Centered Payoff* shows you how to manage stresses, avoid hazards and take control of your practice's destiny in the coming age of 24/7 patient relationships. Capko and Bisera's field-tested techniques are the ultimate guide for the medical practice that wants to stake its claim as its community's top choice for health care services.

From taking an honest look at your practice—providers, staff, culture, even the facility—to creating a positive culture for success, there's a wealth of knowledge here waiting for you to put into action. If you are a practice leader who is not content to just wait and see what happens next, *The Patient-Centered Payoff* is for you."

ELIZABETH W. WOODCOCK, MBA, FACMPE, CPC
Speaker, Author, Consultant
Woodcock & Associates
Atlanta, Georgia

"Health reform has the potential to fundamentally alter the patient-physician relationship. *The Patient-Centered Payoff: Driving Practice Growth through Image, Culture, and Patient Experience* guides physicians on how to maintain and strengthen their relationships with their patients as their practice environment changes around them. Through case studies and extensive consulting experience, Judy Capko and Cheryl Bisera's straightforward and practical style provides common sense ways for both primary care doctors and specialists to successfully navigate the turbulent health care times ahead."

KEVIN PHO, MD
Founder and Editor, KevinMD.com
Co-author of *Establishing, Managing, and Protecting Your Online Reputation: A Social Media Guide for Physicians and Medical Practices*
Nashua, NH

"Judy Capko has done it again. This book, with co-author Cheryl Bisera, offers practical, helpful strategies for successful patient retention. The use of case studies and real life experiences highlight what you can do, starting today, to improve your patient satisfaction scores."

OWEN DAHL, MBA

Owen Dahl Consulting and MGMA Consultant
Author, *Think Business! Medical Practice Quality, Efficiency, Profits*
The Woodlands, TX

"The new book, by Judy Capko and Cheryl Bisera, *The Patient-Centered Payoff: Driving Practice Growth Through Image, Culture, and Patient Experience* is an insightful, yet accurate look at today's medical practice environment. Each chapter builds upon itself with many examples that can help any practice, large or small, achieve better patient satisfaction and consequently more patients. The chapter entitled "Twenty-One Things You Can Do Now (Without Breaking the Bank)" has helped our practice complete an assessment and make some minor changes that have resulted in marked differences in patient satisfaction. It has been eye-opening to the physicians in the practice how a few small gestures to a patient have made such a positive impact without increasing overhead at all."

KIMBERLY WEIS AVERY, MBA, JD

Administrator and General Counsel
Mid-South Pulmonary Specialists, PC
Memphis, TN

"*The Patient-Centered Payoff: Driving Practice Growth Through Image, Culture, and Patient Experience* is an enjoyable read for practice administrators and other healthcare professionals seeking to enhance their medical practice through the patient experience. This book provides recommendations and ideas that are practical and patient-centered, as opposed to bottom-line solutions that do not consider the impact on the patient's experience or satisfaction with the service. I personally appreciate the multiple references on how to engage staff. Eliciting ideas from all of the members of the patient care team is a key success factor that is often overlooked."

SUADA HUSIC, MA, CPC

Training Manager
Weill Cornell Physician Organization
New York, NY

"One of the greatest challenges of owning a medical practice is not only do you need to be a great doctor, you must also be a great business person. This requires a deep understanding of your audience—your patients. Whether you're just starting out or have been practicing a long time, this is a must read to keep your medical practice relevant in an ever changing health care environment."

DONNELLY WILKES, MD
Wilkes Family Medicine
Newbury Park, CA

"If physicians and business managers read and follow the advice provided by Judy Capko and Cheryl Bisera in *The Patient Centered Payoff* they can build a patient culture that will help position their practice for the future. There are so many factors that drive practice growth and not many books complete the picture in a way that is easily understood—this book does.

It really does take a village to improve all aspects that affect practice growth, harmony within the practice, and patient confidence. With this book, one can easily identify areas that need improvement, set goals, and create close to perfect conditions for operating a successful practice. And everyone in the office can participate in this change. Kudos to the authors for turning not-so-interesting topics into content that is sexy and exciting!"

CYNDEE WESTON, CPC, CMC, CMR
Executive Director
American Medical Billing Association (AMBA)
Davis, OK

"*The Patient-Centered Payoff: Driving Practice Growth through Image, Culture and Patient Experience* provides the roadmap needed to thrive in today's changing medical practice landscape. I can't tell you the number of times I have walked into a practice only to be amazed at the mixed messages that the practice atmosphere, staff & communication give.

Practices that understand the interrelationship between culture, branding and staff morale in supporting the patient experience will be better suited to meet the needs of patients and will have better outcomes as a result. I highly recommend this book"

PETER BLANCHARD, MHL
Director of Network Development
Bethany Healthcare Services
Dallas, TX

"Judy Capko and Cheryl Bisera have developed a manual for success in today's rapidly changing healthcare environment. The authors have performed a thorough H&P (history and physical) and differential diagnosis of the attitudes that contribute to poor healthcare outcomes. This prescription works because it is a holistic approach that injects commonsense back into the process of delivering care for better health.

Through their case studies, they have chronicled that the most effective activities involve a simple change in attitude—being patient-centric. This is a revelation and an inexpensive way to begin to repair our broken healthcare system."

DEBBIE DONOVAN

Director of Communications and Corporate Identity
EndoGastric Solutions
Mountain View, CA

"Judy and Cheryl have created a great work. As physicians we are always focused on quality. What we sometimes forget is that we are also in a service industry. Our job is to not only ensure high quality but excellent patient service as well. This book captures this element perfectly and could not be timelier. It is well written and very practical. It should be required reading for all new doctors."

A.H. (TREY) CHANDLER, III MD

Carolina Cardiology Consultants
Division Chief of Cardiology, Greenville Health System
Greenville, SC

"Transform good patient encounters in your practice to experiences that your patients will rave about to their friends, family and on-line . . . this book tells you how.

Improving patient satisfaction is good for a practice in a fee-for-service environment (more referrals, loyal patients) and in an era of shared savings and Accountable Care Organizations (better ratings, higher pay). Use the strategies in this book to accomplish higher ratings.

Only buy this book if you want your patients to refer other patients, if you hope to improve your patient satisfaction and engagement ratings, if you are determined to feel proud of the work you and your staff do every day, and if you want your competitors to ask, "How do they do it?"

BETSY NICOLETTI, MS, CPC

Founder, www.Codapedia.com
Springfield, VT

THE
Patient-
Centered
Payoff

DRIVING PRACTICE GROWTH
THROUGH IMAGE, CULTURE, AND
PATIENT EXPERIENCE

JUDY CAPKO
CHERYL BISERA

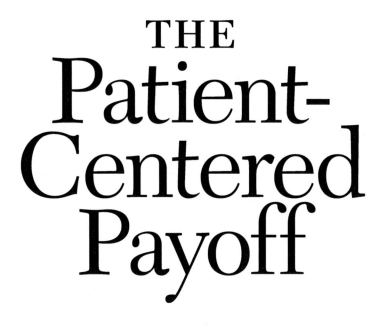

GREENBRANCH
PUBLISHING

To Kyle at the Acorn
Thanks for your interest!

2014

CONTENTS

ACKNOWLEDGMENTS

We feel honored to be given this opportunity to share our knowledge, experience, and passion regarding what it means to be patient centered and the steps that can be taken to strengthen physicians' relationships with their patients, improving the healthcare environment and outcomes for the benefit of both patients and healthcare professionals.

Our thanks to Nancy Collins of Greenbranch Publishing for believing in us, understanding the importance of this topic, and her incredible guidance as we prepared the manuscript. We appreciate all the members of the Greenbranch team, who are professional, dependable, flexible, and a pleasure to work with. We are particularly grateful for the talents of our gifted copy editor, Karen Doyle, who kept us on track and ensured our ideas were expressed clearly. Nancy and Karen, you helped us create the book we dreamed of.

We are grateful to Laurie Morgan, MBA, of Capko & Company in San Francisco for sharing in Chapter 4 her hands-on understanding of social media opportunities for physicians and healthcare organizations. We are also grateful to architect and colleague Larry Brooks, AIA, the owner of Practice Flow Solutions in Atlanta, for sharing in Chapter 9 his wealth of experience and expertise with our readers. We thank you both for your generous contribution from which our readers will gain so much.

We are thankful for the contributions of the physicians, allied healthcare staff, and hospitals that are discussed in the case studies throughout the book, as well as for the patients and healthcare professionals who provided the "Voices from the Field" in Chapter 10. Although some of them remain anonymous, these case studies and testimonials are real and provide valuable insight from first-hand experiences, some of which are shared from deeply personal and painful incidents. We never take for granted the value of these shared experiences and the honor of working side by side with our clients to help improve their patients' experience and the efficiency and profitability of their practice, whether it be through marketing or management consulting.

We acknowledge physicians everywhere that spend many years and make large financial and personal investments in order to practice medicine, a respected and often sacrificial profession. We applaud America for the freedom it affords and for a healthcare system with the highest level of innovation and technology—a country filled with physicians and medical personnel dedicated to serving people of every economic position so that all of us can enjoy healthier lives.

Additional behind-the-scenes expertise was provided by Tim Schmidt, a creative genius with no time but a generous heart; Kristin Borg of Borg Design Group, Inc.; Rena Petrello of Rena Petrello Photography; and Dennis Ricci of Compelling StorySeller. Your professionalism, feedback and generosity are much appreciated.

Our families deserve our gratitude as they listened to our kitchen-table talks about "the book," overheard our sometimes-heated debates, and were willing to find their next meal without our help when we were completely buried in our writing. They were both patient and supportive, even when we were exasperated! One of those kitchen-table discussions resulted in the final title of this book, and we believe it is perfect. For in the end, we hope that every reader will embrace a patient-centered culture and reap the many Patient-Centered Payoffs!

ABOUT THE AUTHORS

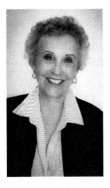 **Judy Capko** is the founder of Capko & Company, www.capko.com, a national healthcare management and marketing consulting firm. She specializes in medical practice operations and practice-building techniques, and focuses on maximizing resources, building patient-centered strategies, and valuing staff contribution. Judy believes we achieve our greatest results by raising others up.

Thousands of physicians and administrators have benefited from her advice and innovative, energetic approach to organizational management and strategic planning for more than 30 years.

Judy is the author of three popular books with Greenbranch Publishing: *Secrets of the Best-Run Practices,* 2005; *Take Back Time—Bringing Time Management to Medicine,* 2002; and *Secrets of the Best-Run Practices,* second edition, 2010. She has been published in more than 50 prestigious national medical journals. She has also written articles for the *Journal of Medical Practice Management®, Urology Times, Eye World, Repertoire, Physicians Practice,* and *Practice Link.*

She is internationally recognized in her field, working with practices both large and small, as well as with major academic faculty practices from coast to coast. She is a popular presenter and keynote speaker for major healthcare conferences and has been a featured presenter at Pri-Med, MGMA, PAHCOM, health plan and health system conferences, national specialty associations, regional medical societies and healthcare executive summits, and corporate healthcare conferences.

Judy and her husband, Joe, live in the Conejo Valley, a beautiful southern California inland coastal community. They have three adult children and eight treasured grandchildren. Judy can be reached at judy@capko.com.

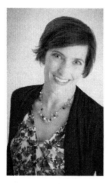

Cheryl Bisera is an author, a speaker, and the founder and leader of Cheryl Bisera Consulting, an image-development and marketing firm focused on the healthcare industry. Her firm's key differentiators are attention to internal marketing, practice branding, and patient experience training. She also provides marketing planning guidance and support, image marketing, and branding services. Cheryl firmly believes that marketing is not only an external activity, but it's also the influence every staff member has on each patient's experience and perception of the practice or healthcare organization.

Her client-specific programs build the practice image while strengthening physician-patient relationships through physician and staff communication programs, mystery guest assessments, and strategies to improve the patient experience. The firm also works with companies that service healthcare professionals by developing marketing and educational programs to help its physician clients succeed in growing new service lines.

A passion for excellence in developing the patient experience and practice image has earned Cheryl impressive testimonials from clients. She speaks for regional medical management organizations and conducts customer-service workshops and training sessions for her clients. She has been published in leading industry journals, including *Podiatry Management, Physician Magazine,* and the *Journal of Medical Practice Management®.* She has also been featured on the popular blog KevinMD.

Cheryl and her husband, Jerrold, are raising their three spirited daughters in Newbury Park, a picturesque southern California community where they enjoy an active lifestyle that includes giving back to their schools, church, and community. Cheryl can be reached at cherylbisera@gmail.com.

Introduction

The inspiration for this book comes from the authors' professional experiences providing management and marketing consulting services for physicians and healthcare organizations around the country and helping these entities adapt to the business challenges they face in a changing healthcare environment. These changes have influenced the attitudes and expectations of the healthcare industry, the government, payers, and consumers. Although there may be some generalization, most readers will be able to relate much of this material to their own personal experiences and work environment, whether they are in a medical practice, diagnostic center, or hospital. For practical purposes, the majority of *The Patient-Centered Payoff* will focus on the medical practice, but it will also provide glimpses into a prestigious hospital, hospital-owned medical practices, an ambulatory surgery center, and a nationally acclaimed children's hospital.

The patient-centered movement promotes a culture of care that is respectful of and responsive to individual patient preferences and needs, and ensures that patient values guide all clinical decisions. A major strategy to accomplish this is strengthening the relationship between physicians and patients, resulting in shared decision-making that improves compliance and results in better population health management.

A TIMELY BOOK

We believe this book is timely and offers valuable information about healthcare reform's intentions to focus on a more patient-centric healthcare system and financially reward physicians based on data intended to measure communication with patients, shared decision-making, and improved patient outcomes.

This book discusses everything from what you can do to provide a better patient experience to how you will benefit from doing so. It also provides information about how the patient-centered movement has evolved, the motivation and goals that drive it, and the financial incentives that are being offered to physicians that succeed in meeting certain patient-centered performance metrics. It outlines practical steps healthcare professionals can take to ensure that their organization is moving in the right direction and reaping the benefits of being patient-centric.

BOOK OVERVIEW

There are three distinct parts to this book that provide detailed information about how these elements affect medical practices and health systems. These key organizational components are:

1. Image;
2. Culture; and
3. The patient experience.

Chapter 1 is all about being best; the factors that form a patient's opinion and what makes patients feel valued by their physician. It discusses how the future of being best will focus on being more patient-centered. Chapter 2 looks at how costly it is to have unhappy patients and what it means to you not only now but in the future. It's time to end the unhappiness epidemic in healthcare! In Chapter 3, we talk about an identity crisis and steps you can take to ensure that your identity and brand are consistent.

Technology has influenced how you practice your profession and how your patients rate you and share their ratings with the rest of the world. Chapter 4, The 24 x 7 Patient Relationship by contributing author Laurie Morgan of Capko & Company, will bring you up to date on social media's influence on your business. It is real, it is powerful, and the more you know about it, the more prepared you will be to live in the world of technology and put technology to work for you.

Chapter 5 is the beginning of your journey into understanding your organizational culture. It contains case studies that showcase what it means to live your mission, how easy it is to create an image collision, and how a hospital's ambitious initiative was launched too soon, among others. In Chapter 6, we focus on the cultural differences that cause a clash when hospitals acquire medical practices and we provide the lessons learned so others can avoid the same problem. Chapter 7 explores the conflicts that exist on the patient-centered journey and how the influences of managed care have affected this voyage. Chapter 8, Mirror, Mirror, presents case studies that may make you take a hard look at your own practice or healthcare facility. It will reveal how you can sometimes get so caught up in what you do that you fail to see things from the patients' perspective. You'll find tips on how to take your practice from average to memorable with just a little effort.

Chapter 9, How Facility Design Impacts the Patient Experience, goes one step further by examining your building and its influence on the patient experience and your efficiency and profitability. It is packed full of information to help you in the design or renovation of a facility so the end result is far more efficient and patient-friendly. This chapter provides recommendations that, if taken, will make your facility work for *you*, not against you, by boosting your ability to be more productive and more profitable. Medical design architect Larry Brooks, AIA, adds valuable content to this chapter. This chapter ends with The Wow Factor, simple things you can do to add visual impact to your practice facility.

Chapter 10, Voices From the Field, is an emotional journey that shares the personal experiences of patients with serious healthcare issues and their interaction with the medical community. These amazing stories, told in the individuals' own words, are honest and reveal the true thoughts, feelings, and vulnerability of the patients and their families. The chapter also profiles several healthcare professionals, offering insight into how they connect with and communicate value to their patients, and why they believe it is so important and the benefits they've reaped in being truly patient-centered. Chapter 11 is full of practical steps to determine what you can put into motion immediately to improve the image, culture, and patient experience in your healthcare business.

The book's final chapter discusses how the patient-centered focus has evolved and why the government has placed additional emphasis on this issue with healthcare reform. We offer leaders steps they can take to set the stage for success, demonstrating their organization's commitment to being patient-centered. This chapter will also discuss financial incentives that are emerging based on meeting specific core measures. We provide an overview of the Patient-Centered Medical Home model and the new recognition program for the Patient-Centered Specialty Practice. In this chapter, you will learn about the standards set to encourage physicians to engage with and strengthen relationships with patients, contributing to shared decision-making, better compliance, and improved patient satisfaction that results in greater financial rewards for physicians and improved health for their patients.

We hope this book will enable you to discover ways to build a best-practice image, embrace a patient-service culture, and create the ultimate patient experience.

CHAPTER 1

Being Best

Physicians certainly have an opinion of their practice and the patient's experience in their office. Unfortunately, they don't typically look at the practice's image or performance from the patient's point of view. They should! It is a factor in complying with smart business practices. Beyond this, insurance payers are now paying physicians based on performance, which means doctors are financially at risk based on patient service. Indeed, it's the opinion of both existing and prospective patients that counts the most. Physicians and their staff have the ability to influence that opinion every single day.

HEALTHCARE CONSULTANTS are typically called into a practice because of problems the practice is experiencing with stagnant or declining revenue, staffing issues, workflow efficiency, partnership issues, or a need to grow the practice, but it is rare for physicians to bring in a consultant because they are concerned about patient satisfaction or the patients' impressions of the practice. There is little concern about the physical appearances or comfort of the office or the staff's appearance and attitude toward patients. This may be because physicians have a distorted picture of what their practice looks like, how it appeals to others, and how the practice rates on the level of service it provides. Perhaps they assume all is well. We hear it during our consulting engagements: "Our patients love us; we give the highest quality of care and service; our service is the best; and we pride ourselves on the quality of our care." In fact, this type of verbiage is often a part of the practice's mission statement. However, these opinions are too often based on *subjective* information or the physician's own biased opinion. Neither of these provides an accurate portrait of the practice. If a practice wants to be considered one of the "best," it needs to have proof that it is one of the top-performing groups—meaning it needs to have *objective* measurements of how patients rate the practice.

Being a *best practice* means being among the top 10%, not simply *above average,* based on objective findings that are statistically tracked and compared with those of other practices. Do you really know how you compare with other practices in your area or in your specialty when it comes to being a patient-centered practice and providing outstanding service? What are the secrets to being best? How can a practice measure such a seemingly intangible and subjective goal? We will explore the answers to these questions, offer additional insights, and hopefully inspire you to become patient-centered and continually employ methods to reach a higher level of patient satisfaction.

PERFORMANCE BENCHMARKS

For years, some of our nation's savviest medical practice executives, managers, and physicians have examined their practice performance by analyzing critical data and comparing their own performance to statistical tracking of similar practices by specialty and size, usually obtained through Medscape (www.medscape.com), the Medical Group Management Association (www.mgma.org), and/or the National Society of Certified Healthcare Business Consultants (www.nschbc.org). These organizations have been collecting benchmarking data for years. This information enables practice management consultants and medical practice administrators and physicians to set goals and better manage performance from year to year in these specific areas:

1. Productivity and efficiency;
2. Profitability and cost control; and
3. Revenue cycle management.

The Fourth Standard

You might be achieving best practice performance based on these factors, but recently a very important fourth standard has been added to the list, and it may be a *game changer*. It is patient satisfaction—giving your patients a high-quality, positive experience that meets and satisfies their needs. It starts with the image of the practice from the patient's perspective on these key factors:

- The look and comfort of the office;
- How respectful and attentive physician and staff are;
- How well everyone communicates;
- Ease of access for visits; and
- Timeliness during the visit.

These are key factors that form patients' opinions and determine whether they feel *valued* by their physician. Every aspect of the image of your practice and the patients' personal experience is reflected in how they rate their level of satisfaction. If patients rate their care and service highly and believe they have been appropriately involved in the clinical decision-making process, they are likely to be more compliant and obtain better clinical outcomes, inevitably proving the case for whether a medical organization or facility is really patient-centered.

> *If a practice wants to be considered one of the "best," it needs to have proof that it is one of the top-performing groups.*

The article "The Ideal Medical Practice Model"[1] presents an interesting model on perfecting the patient experience. It includes a survey based on 50 practices. Twelve of the practices responding were identified as ideal, and 38 were usual. The findings are intriguing and are just one example of how the healthcare industry is placing more importance on how patients rate their experience. This study scored physicians on how patients felt about their care, whether they received exactly what they wanted; the efficiency and organization of the medical office and not wasting the patient's time; the ease of getting care; the level of education provided about their condition; and whether the physician was aware of their emotional needs. The ideal medical practice generally reported better care than the usual care practices. According to the authors, "patient reports of their health care experiences are important because they tend to correlate with patients' clinical outcomes."[1] This certainly would explain the shifting focus on the importance of the patient experience.

When preparing to write this book, we conducted our own patient survey to determine how patients rate their experience with the physician's office on seven key points:

1. Ease of access for visit;
2. Office décor updated and comfortable;

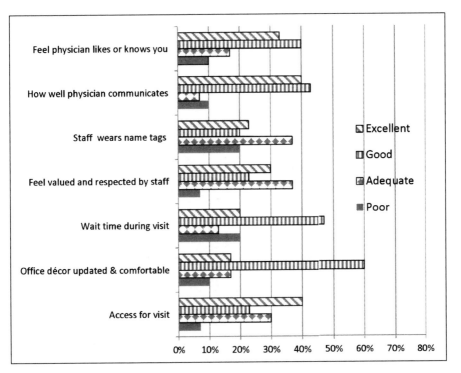

FIGURE 1. Patient satisfaction survey results.

3. Wait time during visit;

4. Feeling valued and respected by staff;

5. Staff wearing name tags;

6. Physician communication; and

7. Feeling that the physician likes or knows the patient.

Patients of more than 10 different specialties from five different metro areas in the country were surveyed. The results (see Figure 1) present some interesting (and some surprising) findings.

The scores on physician communication were impressive with 83% of the respondents rating physicians as excellent or good, with 40% rating their physician as an excellent communicator. When asked if they felt that the physician likes or knows them, 33% rated their physician as excellent. However, 27% of the patients did not feel this way, rating the physician as poor or only adequate, leaving some room for improvement. Regardless, these findings indicate most physicians are succeeding in providing an attentive, respectful interaction with their patients.

Unfortunately, staff did not score as well with making patients feel valued and respected. Only 30% rated staff as excellent, and 23% rated staff as good. Sadly, 37% felt staff performed only adequately, and 7% rated staff as poor in making them feel valued and respected. Additionally, 57% of the surveyed patients also rated staff poorly or only adequate for wearing name tags or introducing themselves to patients. Our own experiences performing mystery visits in medical practices around the country validate these findings.

If patients rate their care and service highly, they are likely to be more compliant.

Physicians almost always introduce themselves and shake hands the first time they meet patients—staff members rarely do, and this includes front office and nursing staff who are the first to interact with new patients in the office. These two scoring elements alone suggest staff members might be less committed to providing patient-centered service than the physicians they work with, might be poorly trained in customer service, or don't understand the importance of their role in the practice and the impact they have on the patient experience. It is crucial that staff members understand the importance of their interaction with patients and receive proper training. Often there is an assumption among the staff that because patients are there to see the doctor, the patients don't care about their interaction with other staff members—staff members feel that they are unimportant members of the team. This kind of thinking can permeate a practice culture and inhibit staff from providing excellent customer service. A commitment to a patient-centered culture begins with physicians and other leaders within the practice. This commitment is demonstrated by how these leaders present and treat staff and whether they invest in training and team-building exercises. A first step can be as simple as dedicating a team meeting to reviewing your mission and discussing how each team member will support it through customer service. The results of our survey indicate that staff members are not communicating or expressing that the patient is valued as well as physicians are. This is further supported in a number of the case studies presented throughout this book.

The scores for access—how quickly a patient can get in to see the doctor—revealed that 40% of the respondents felt access was excellent, and 23% rated access as good. Seven percent of the practices did poorly with appointment access, and 30% were rated only adequate. This suggests that as many as 37% of patients wanting appointments are waiting an unreasonable amount of time to see their physician. This is an important metric because a delay in diagnosis and treatment can cause conditions to worsen and result in poor clinical outcomes, more emergency department visits, and increased healthcare costs. Another time-related issue important to patient satisfaction and well-being is timeliness, which reflects how long a patient waits once he or she arrives for an appointment. In our survey, 20% of the practices were rated excellent and 47% good, recognizing that many practices are efficient with scheduling and patient flow. However, 33% of the practices received a score that indicated they were just adequate or poor in timeliness. If you suspect that your practice is not meeting the access or timeliness needs of your patients, it may be time to call in an expert to evaluate your scheduling patterns, demands for access, and patient flow and provide solutions to these key performance issues.

We believe one of the most interesting findings of the survey is how medical practices are performing with the décor and comfort of the practice. Although only 17% of the practices scored an excellent, an unexpected 60% were rated as good. This is certainly not the case with the many hundreds of practices the authors have visited. We believe at least 50% of practices around the country have reception rooms that look shabby, lack comfort, are not sufficient in size, and often have tattered magazines and reading materials that are not appropriate for their patient demographics. It appears our standards are higher than those of the respondents, who may be more accepting of these issues. We do find that larger practices and health systems that own physician practices, as well as practices that offer elective services, fare much better, with facilities that are polished, fresh, and designed for comfort. This may be because larger systems and aesthetic practices have marketing and service departments that tend to better understand the importance of these issues and have the resources to dedicate to them. The tools found in this book can be applied to both types of organizations as well as smaller practices with limited resources in order to leave a stellar impression on your patients—and reap outstanding ratings.

Most organizations that have conducted patient satisfaction studies in the past have not scored indicators such as first impressions, condition of facility, and staff and physician appearance, and how these matters affect the patient. Determining if you are in the top 10 percentile with the image your practice portrays, understanding patients' perceptions, and learning how patients view the experience in your practice are important, but it is more important that healthcare providers *care enough* to make the changes required to create the ultimate patient experience. We hope this book will help you to understand that patient satisfaction is a game changer for the healthcare industry, and there are no exemptions. Whether you are affiliated with a healthcare system, hospital, surgery center, or medical practice, it is up to each of you to become a winner in this new game—and the clock starts ticking now.

FACING REALITY:
PATIENT SATISFACTION IS A BIG DEAL

Healthcare systems, hospitals, and health plans have been surveying their patients for years. A number of academic faculty practices,
integrated healthcare systems, and larger specialty practices have
contracted with marketing consultants and independent surveyors
to gather information to rate their facilities' performance. Because
of this, they are better prepared to withstand the changes that will
influence how they will be paid with healthcare reform, which will
reward providers that score well with satisfying patients' needs both
in and out of the hospital.

The Centers for Medicare & Medicaid Services (CMS) will reduce its
payments for hospitals by 1% or an estimated $963 million for this
fiscal year (2013).[2] It will then distribute the money to those hospitals with high scores on a varied matrix, and patient satisfaction
surveys will make up 30% of that score. By 2017, the withholding will
double to 2%. Hospitals and major academic centers are scrutinizing
physician behavior, recognizing it has tremendous influence on their
satisfaction scores—and therefore their bottom line.

A commitment to a patient-centered culture
begins with physicians and other leaders
within the practice.

According to Kevin B. O'Reilly, the University of Wisconsin (UW)
Medical Foundation recently created a new compensation plan for the
primary care physicians in the UW faculty.[3] This compensation plan
offers a 5% increase in pay based on a set of performance measures,
including patient satisfaction. UW is just one of many big industry
players that are incentivizing doctors, according to an October 2011
report by The Hay Group, a Philadelphia-based management consulting firm.[3]

Nearly two-thirds of hospitals, health systems, and large physician groups have annual incentive plans for doctors, according to the Hay Group report. Sixty-two percent of these organizations use patient satisfaction metrics as a factor, up from 43% in 2010, said the survey of 182 healthcare organizations covering physicians in 144 medical specialties. Many set base pay lower and require doctors to meet performance metrics to earn hefty incentive pay, according to O'Reilly.

We have conducted hundreds of practice assessments during the past 25 years. During these engagements, we discovered a number of healthcare systems, larger medical practices, and academic faculty practices that were conducting patient satisfaction surveys. However, some of them were struggling to achieve their performance improvement goals. In fact in some cases, this was the very reason they sought our services. There is often a gap between the administrative management's understanding of the need to measure patient satisfaction and that of the physicians and staff, who may have only a vague understanding of why these surveys are necessary.

Many healthcare provider groups have great difficulty in making the cultural shift that creates a patient-centered environment. Often they struggle to change the attitudes and behaviors of physicians in order to improve the patient experience. This suggests that the very people caring for and interacting with patients the most are not taking patient satisfaction as seriously as other areas of performance. Furthermore, this supports the need to adapt physician compensation plans to financially reward physicians that succeed at creating a better patient experience.

Our experience working with smaller practices—those with fewer than 20 physicians—has been quite different. Most of them make broad assumptions that their patients are happy and, therefore, see no need to conduct surveys. They typically tell us that their patients are satisfied, and they tout the quality of service their practice provides, even though there are no reliable, unbiased data to support this belief. Conducting patient surveys would equip these smaller practices with objective findings, making it possible to implement changes that could result in exponential growth, stellar reviews, and validation of a job well done.

In the past, with finances and operational efficiency being the drivers of profitability, executive healthcare management teams gave these factors far more attention than patient satisfaction. That is changing as pay for performance brings patient satisfaction into the financial arena.

In the proposed 2013 Medicare physician fee schedule, CMS outlined plans to include patient satisfaction survey results for group practices participating in the Physician Quality Reporting System on the Physician Compare Web site no sooner than 2014. Starting in 2013, physicians who do not report enough quality metrics to CMS will see a 1.5% Medicare pay cut in 2015, which will rise to 2% in 2016 and beyond.

These changes validate the need for physicians and healthcare executives to be patient-centered and to instill this viewpoint into their practice culture through example. In other words, it is your job to make this cultural shift from within in order to succeed and withstand the winds of change.

PATIENT-CENTERED, NOT PATIENT-LED, HEALTHCARE

In a recent University of California, Davis study of more than 50,000 adults, an *inverse* relationship between patient satisfaction scores and health outcomes surfaced.[4] Surprisingly, in this study, those most satisfied with their healthcare providers were, on average, *sicker* than their less satisfied counterparts. Additionally, though perhaps not as surprising, healthcare costs were about 9% higher for these most satisfied patients.

Among possible explanations is that physicians, motivated in part by physician compensation structures that consider patient satisfaction, may stray from standard treatments to meet patient expectations. Though an increase in tests and procedures may satisfy a patient who believes *more is better*, clinical outcomes can suffer when patients are exposed to the risks of unnecessary treatments.

> *Many small practices make broad assumptions that their patients are happy and, therefore, see no need to conduct surveys.*

This study and our experience call into question the value of very broad measures of patient satisfaction (i.e., "How satisfied are you overall?"), because patients are notorious for confusing bedside manner with the quality of clinical care.

The implications of this study may be far-reaching, but enterprising providers can take simple steps to educate their patients, preferably long before they see them in the exam room. With e-mail and social media making communication easier and less expensive, creating simple and regular communications can help inform patients of the risks and costs of unnecessary tests and treatments. Being assured that you have their best interest in mind, and are not holding out for any other reason, can put patients at ease and help them to more readily accept your recommendations in spite of feeling anxious about their health.

Though studies have indicated payers and large health organizations generally accept that improved communication and a patient-centered environment is a win-win-win for payers, patients, and providers, it is critical that physicians maintain their ethics and integrity and not succumb to a patient's unreasonable demands for clinical treatment that is not appropriate. You can win high satisfaction ratings by providing a stellar patient experience without compromising your expertise and recommendations—after all, patients come to *you* for that!

MAKE THE COMMITMENT

When a health system, hospital, ambulatory surgery center, or medical practice measures performance, it creates a baseline with which it can compare its business to similar organizations. It can then set goals and benchmarks for improvement.

Your commitment to becoming a better performing practice (in regard to the patient experience) begins with an honest look at your own patient satisfaction report card and, much like looking at practice finances, taking the report seriously.

On the quest to improving patient satisfaction, it is important to remember that the results of patient surveys are influenced by the level of commitment, consistency, and accountability within the organization. By continuing to raise the bar each year, an average-performing practice can obtain amazing results and reap the rewards of high patient satisfaction and meaningful care partnerships. There is much to be gained by being among the best.

THE PAYOFF

Believing you are among the best practices is insignificant if, in fact, your patients don't agree. Understanding what patients really think and feel is the beginning of a journey that can result in an ideal doctor-patient relationship where patients feel valued, become loyal referrers, and are more compliant.

References

1. Moore GL, Wasson JH. The ideal medical practice model: improving efficiency, quality and the doctor-patient relationship. *Fam Pract Manag.* 2007;14(8):20-24; www.aafp.org/fpm/2007/0900/p20.html.

2. Adamy J. U.S. ties hospital payment to making patients happy. *Wall Street Journal.* October 14, 2012; http://online.wsj.com/article/SB100008723963904438903045780102641560731 32.html.

3. O'Reilly KB. Patient satisfaction: when a doctor's judgment risks a poor rating. amednews.com. November 26, 2012; www.amednews.com/article/20121126/profession/311269934/4/.

4. Falkenberg K. Why rating doctors is bad for your health. *Forbes.* January 21, 2013; www.forbes.com/sites/kaifalkenberg/2013/01/02/why-rating-your-doctor-is-bad-for-your-health/.

CHAPTER 2

Unhappy Patients Are Costly

Unhappy patients: every practice has them. Maybe you believe you have very few, or perhaps you're reading this because you know you have too many. Unhappy patients are sometimes sneaky; quietly disappearing so that you never knew they were, well, unhappy. More than 90%[1] will not say anything; they will simply go away and vow never to do business with you again. They may not tell you why they left, but they will tell people in their sphere of influence, and that should be of grave concern to you.

IT'S THE SNEAKY (QUIET) PATIENTS that cost you the most and give you the least opportunity to improve. Are unhappy patients an unavoidable nuisance that you and your staff usher through the system and breathe a sigh of relief once they leave, or are they something far more indicative of why your practice isn't meeting its potential? Any sigh of relief when they walk out the door is misguided because *that's* when an unhappy patient begins to drain your practice of potential revenue.

Physicians go to school for umpteen years, scratch away at their education debt, work long hours trying to fix other people's often complex problems, and *now* they have to worry about how those patients might hurt the practice's bottom line if the physicians look at them the wrong way? It may sound absurd and over-reactive at first, but the truth is that patients are a barometer for the quality of care and service they receive. It's not just potential patients who are paying attention to "unhappy patients," payers are too. Facing the demands of today's changing marketplace is your path to success. Charles Darwin said, "It's not the strongest of the species that survives, nor the most intelligent, but the one most responsive to change"—so it is in your medical practice.

PAY FOR PERFORMANCE

Next year, nearly one billion dollars in payments to hospitals will be based partially on patient satisfaction, this being determined by a Centers for Medicare & Medicaid Services' survey administered to patients. Hospitals that score high with patients will receive bonus payments, those with low scores will lose money. This program is part of a much broader pay-for-performance system built into the healthcare overhaul that will affect future payments to physicians. Times are changing, and payers are looking for new ways to measure care and patient experiences. The result is an increased focus on the patient's overall experience and financial accountability of providers, be it reward or penalty.

It may seem unreasonable, being asked to focus on these nonclinical issues. But studies show a strong correlation between patient satisfaction and patient compliance, ultimately resulting in improved outcomes. You *can* succeed on the customer service front while maintaining your clinical integrity and thriving financially—your first step was picking up this book!

THE *REAL* COST OF ATTRITION

When patients quietly change physicians and you simply don't see them again, you've lost money. You've not only lost the revenue from their visits, but the potential visits of their extended family. You've also lost potential revenue from the business of their friends, neighbors, and coworkers who would have given considerable weight to the answer to this question, "Who do you see for _____?" when they ask your former patients next week, next month, or next year. How will you attract patients to make up for attrition and at what cost?

> *Times are changing, and payers are looking for new ways to measure care and patient experiences.*

Some physicians maintain that the demand for their services is so great that an unhappy patient leaving the practice has no significant impact. In reality, even if this patient never participated in a survey conducted by one of your insurance payers, there is a high *internal* cost to attrition.

To begin with, there is the cost of time and resources required to create and maintain visibility for your practice. This includes contracting to be on an insurance plan's provider list and marketing—which when done right will cost you time, money, and effort. Next is the cost of resources to query and schedule a new patient, and gather and record data in preparation for the patient's visit. Then, of course, the expense of time and resources to integrate a new patient into the practice and gather historical clinical data, and time spent face-to-face. For these reasons, new patient visits are generally less profitable than subsequent follow-up or existing patient visits. Studies have shown that it costs approximately five times more to obtain a new customer than to retain an existing one.[2] It takes subsequent visits to begin to recoup the costs of obtaining and setting up a new patient in your system. If a new patient is discontented, there may not be a subsequent visit. Unhappy patients lead to attrition, attrition is costly, and therefore unhappy patients are costly.

YOUR REPUTATION IS AT STAKE

When patients leave your practice, you may not even know that they had a bad experience until it's too late. The digital age has empowered consumers to voice their opinions and rate their experiences online, reaching hundreds or even thousands of potential new customers. Potential patients can "check you out" by reading posts from your patients on review sites such as Healthgrades.com, Yelp.com, and Vitals.com. A personal testimony is powerful and has great influence on whether or not a shopping patient will take the next step toward choosing you as his or her physician. Unfortunately, it's the unhappy customers that are most motivated to post, and they have little at stake for publically slamming you. (In Chapter 4, we present the how-tos of managing your online reputation.)

Reputation damage caused by unhappy patients can quickly destroy the practice you worked so hard to build and cause economic disaster you may never be able to overcome. Warren Buffett once said, "It takes 20 years to build a reputation and five minutes to ruin it. If you think about that, you'll do things differently."[3] Consider these statistics[4]:

- For every customer who bothers to complain, there are 26 others that remain silent.
- A *dissatisfied* customer will tell 9 to 15 people about it, 13% of them will tell 20 people about their experience.

It is important to recognize that patient satisfaction, or lack thereof, is going to affect your bottom line—reputation is an irreplaceable commodity.

NONCOMPLIANT PATIENTS HURT THE PRACTICE

Not every patient is going to be compliant, that's a given; but when a patient feels known and valued by his or her physician and the practice, chances are the patient *will* be compliant. Developing strong relationships and high levels of patient satisfaction can lead to improved communication and compliance, ultimately leading to improved outcomes. Patients who don't feel connected, valued, or personally known by their physician are more likely to stop listening to the physician, become noncompliant, and take their medical care into their own hands.

If a new patient is discontented, there may not be a subsequent visit.

Noncompliant patients don't follow your treatment plan, don't keep their appointments, and/or don't take their medications as prescribed. They are frustrating for everyone in the practice and difficult to manage—they can be downright annoying, and their expectations can be unrealistic. Sometimes they are unhappy long before they stop following your treatment regimen and stop giving you the respect you and your staff deserve. Everyone in the practice may know them as "high-maintenance patients" that take up far more time than the average patient; calling frequently, demanding to get an appointment immediately, and asking for medications and testing that the physician deems inappropriate. These types of patients, despite their lack of compliance, are more likely to be the ones that threaten to sue you, switch physicians, and disparage your reputation in the community. There is a high price to pay for noncompliant patients: frustration, an unpleasant work environment, the cost of resources to manage them, and the potential damage to your reputation.

> *Noncompliant patients represent significant cost for your medical practice.*

This lack of respect and noncompliance are costly in many ways beyond the interaction with your practice (Figure 1). It is not uncommon for noncompliant patients to ignore deteriorating health conditions and further compromise their health. Such patients end up in the emergency department, sometimes resulting in extensive, costly diagnostic studies and hospitalization. The costs of these noncompliant patients place further burden on our healthcare system and are under scrutiny by the government and private health insurance plans, resulting in the emergence of the Patient-Centered Medical Home. Measuring and improving clinical outcomes is a strategy within healthcare reform aimed at keeping patients healthier, coordinating care among providers, getting sick patients better quicker, educating patients, and encouraging healthy lifestyles with the ultimate goal of reducing the cost of healthcare. Physicians play a vital role in accomplishing these goals by marrying their clinical skills with stronger patient-physician relationships built on trust and respect.

The intent of a patient-centered practice is to create a better health partnership between healthcare providers and their patients.

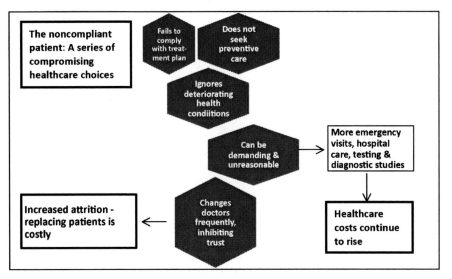

FIGURE 1. Costs of noncompliant patients.

THE UNHAPPINESS EPIDEMIC

There's been an outbreak of unhappiness in your practice—disgruntled patients, stressed-out employees, and burned-out physicians. If you ask who had "the bug" first, each person points to someone else. Symptoms are distinct: patients grumble as they reluctantly hand over their copays, staff members have to resist the temptation to close *and lock* the glass window at the check-in desk, and physicians roll their eyes upon exiting an exam room. It's nearly impossible to find the first victim and determine how it spread, but there is no question that a terrible case of unhappiness has come to rest in your practice and there is no known cure—or is there?

When the unhappiness virus hits, it costs your practice in all kinds of ways you might not have considered. Unhappy patients affect the job satisfaction of every staff member. Their complaints, disrespect, and ingratitude rob employees of a pleasant work environment. Employees want to feel good about their job, with a sense of purpose and accomplishment at the end of the day. Good employees that recognize the lack of support and accountability to deliver stellar patient care will not stay. The cost is often high turnover and a poorly performing staff (that feel there is nothing to aspire to), more demanding patients, and burned out providers—all of which cost your practice time, money, and effort.

Patients don't enjoy being grumpy; they want great service and to thank you for it. When respect is extended to the patient, surely it will be reaped in loyalty, referrals, and compliance. When service is lacking, you may be attracting only patients that feel they *have* to come to you. Their lack of enthusiasm is evident after a long wait time and grumbled instructions by your staff. Their reaction only adds to the impression of them that your staff members have: patients are a necessary evil, a nuisance they must "put up with." An inefficient office with poor customer service is not a fun place to work; as you can see, no one is happy in this scenario.

There is a cure, even a vaccine, to stave off this practice culture that steals job-fulfillment, money, time, and reputation. It begins with the belief that you *can*, and the knowledge of *how*—both of which we hope to empower you with between the pages of this book. You *can* improve the patient experience, boost your reputation, and enjoy a more fulfilling and profitable career!

THE PAYOFF

Keeping patients happy is good for the patients and good for the practice. A patient that is happy with his or her healthcare experience is more cooperative and has better outcomes, resulting in improved ratings, better reimbursement, and reduced risk for healthcare providers.

References

1. Zaibak O. 20 Customer Service Statistics for 2011. Customer 1. October 13, 2010; www.customer1.com/blog/customer-service-statistics.
2. MillerJB, with Brown PB. *The Corporate Coach*. New York: St. Martin's Press, May 1993,
3. Tuttle B. Warren Buffett's boring, brilliant wisdom. *Time*. March 1, 2010; http://business.time.com/2010/03/01/warren-buffetts-boring-brilliant-wisdom/.
4. Customer Service Facts. Customer Service Manager.com. www.customerservicemanager.com/customer-service-facts.htm.

CHAPTER 3

From Identity Crisis to Brand Recognition

Today's physician, whether employed by a large academic faculty practice or health system, a solo practitioner, or a partner in private practice, is required to master skills that entail applying business principles to the business of medicine and getting involved in efforts to improve the future of medicine. This is in addition to meeting ever-changing criteria to ensure optimal reimbursements, and staying on top of the latest technology and research in his or her specialty. With all these changes and demands, physicians, healthcare delivery systems, or practices can easily lose sight of what makes them unique; the specific focus and values that drive them, and how to differentiate themselves in the eyes of patients. In some instances, physicians and practices are treading so feverishly to keep their heads above water that they have no idea how they fit into the competitive landscape, thus creating an "identity crisis."

HOW CAN PHYSICIANS and healthcare systems identify their unique qualities, define their mission and market position, and then communicate and practice their mission consistently in order to build credibility, loyalty, and overall success? To successfully do this, you must know, communicate, and live up to your desired identity in a way that is patient-centered in every sense of the word. In the business world, it's called branding; and these days, it's vital to thriving in a competitive marketplace.

Within the pages of this book, you will find strategies to implement in order to meet patients' nonmedical needs and exceed patients' expectations in ways that will keep them coming back. But truly, before you can exceed expectations, before you can create awareness, before you can successfully get all your employees aligned on a patient-centered team, you must grasp who you are as a physician, as a practice, or as a hospital or other healthcare business. Then you must define it in patient-centered terms, thus answering the question for your patients, "Why should I choose you?" and for your staff, "Why are we here?"

Certainly an academic physician choosing to delve into research in the hope of finding the next great cure has a mission that is different from a primary care physician in a rural community, an orthopaedic surgeon specializing in sports medicine for an NFL team, an emergency department physician, or a medical director for a large insurance plan that has the power to set policy that will affect the future of medical practices around the country. Who are you, and what do you *really* want to achieve as a physician? Few physicians practicing medicine today give this the thought it deserves, but clearly understanding your purpose and defining your mission will empower you. It will influence the way you practice medicine and the service and attention given to your patients by your staff.

CREATE A MISSION STATEMENT

A mission statement is a short, descriptive phrase or sentence that is easy to remember and illustrates the practice's goals and purpose, as defined by the owners. It is about deciding what is important to you and your practice. Its simplicity gives it strength, but it is only as strong as the commitment you make. So be cautious and thoughtful in developing your mission statement. Make sure you can stand by it over time. For example, saying your mission is to *"Provide the best radiation oncology treatment in the community"* might be hard to prove or fulfill, but stating your mission is to *"Provide innovative solutions in radiation oncology"* may be reasonable if you are teaching fellows at a university medical center and participating in clinical trials.

When we help practices develop their mission statement, we often will collaborate with the entire team. Once the mission statement is established, we work with the practice to determine what strategies will be implemented to fulfill the mission. Getting the buy-in of your staff members is essential because they are the ones who must deliver on the mission every day with every patient. The purpose of your mission statement is to define for your staff, patients, and community why your practice exists, using simple, easy-to-grasp terms. Once it is created, it serves as an important tool to guide future strategic business decisions, ensuring your actions fulfill the mission and never compromise your purpose.

EXPRESS IT WITH CONVICTION

Once you have a mission statement, everyone in the practice should know it. One of our pet peeves is asking practice staff members if they have a practice mission statement only to discover that some employees don't know if there is one, and others know there is one but don't remember what it says. Your mission statement has no value if the practice doesn't live it, and employees can't live it if they don't know what it is. No matter how meaningful your mission statement is to you, it rings hollow to your patients if it's not lived out in every interaction they have with your practice. In Chapter 5, we delve into the importance of *living up to* your mission statement. Once you're doing that, display it prominently in the reception room and staff lounge. State it on the practice Web site and appropriate collateral materials. You need to shout it from the rooftops, burn it into memory, and express it with pride and conviction.

BRANDING

After defining who you are, professionally speaking, and the mission that drives your practice, it's time to leverage a practice identity to appeal to existing patients and attract the type of patients you want. Begin by asking who your target market is and what your "style" or "personality" is, as a practice. Is your practice the fun, casual pediatric practice that wants every child and teen to feel they're in a practice environment designed for them? Perhaps it's a cosmetic dermatology practice wanting to attract patients for services that might otherwise be sought at a medical spa. Everything from your practice name to your logo, Web site, messaging, and even staff uniforms and office décor needs to communicate a distinct image to your target market—the patients you wish to attract and retain.

LOGO

A picture is worth a thousand words; and in the case of your logo, a thousand words you're going to be repeating over and over for many years in many places. For this reason, it's worth taking the time and money to do it right. If your mission is to make kids smile, your logo should be happy and something easily understood by your patients. And if your target patients are children, you must appeal to their parents who bring them to the practice. A logo must evoke a sense of comfort, friendliness, and positive affirmations. Your logo needs to be somewhat timeless, allowing for changes in society and demographics. It also needs to be broad enough to allow for any growth you foresee in the near future (not limiting you should you add services), communicate credibility and professionalism, and be "clean."

A clean logo is one that is not complex and is easy to recognize; works in black and white just as well as in color; and is flexible— you can use it on a pen, your Web site, a t-shirt or a give-away bag. Further, your logo should be able to stand alone and still visually communicate what your services entail without the support of copy and photography.

Leverage your practice identity to appeal to existing patients and attract the type of patients you want.

Surely you don't recommend that your patients perform their own procedures or diagnose themselves, they don't have the proper training and experience. Neither should you consider yourself an expert in design and branding. A healthcare marketing expert can guide the creative process, collaborating with a designer while considering your goals and your target patients. A competent graphic designer will design a style board that reflects your brand. This includes your logo, a color palette, typography (fonts), graphic elements, and stylized photography. This style board becomes a guideline for all your other corporate collateral. Maintaining consistency throughout all your marketing pieces communicates a sense of organization, experience, and dependability. The style board can be referred to for Web design and even help guide décor and uniform decisions. A professional copywriter or marketing consultant can assist in writing a tagline and some key words to be used repeatedly in future copy. Let a professional's creativity and skill bring your desired image to a level you never could accomplish on your own.

We've worked with many physicians whose lead in this process resulted in disastrous design. From the physician's perspective, the designs—be it logo, Web site, or messaging—were "slick," "creative," and invoked positive emotions, *for them*. Physicians' bias and lack of expertise in this area can prevent them from recognizing that a design is unprofessional, dated, overly clinical, too complex, or even disturbing in the eyes of their patients. Often medical specialists are so enamored with the body part they focused on in their fellowship that they believe it would be best to feature this body part, in logo form, on their business cards, brochures, and Web site.

Your patients are not in love with your specialty, may cringe at the thought of what their insides look like, and do not want to be thought of as an anatomical body part or condition. They don't want to be reminded that there may be something wrong with this part of their body. The following case study is a perfect example of a practice falling short in communicating its strengths and unique qualities, so much so that its branding was de-marketing this practice.

CASE STUDY
Design Disaster Diverted

Gilbert Simoni, MD, a talented gastroenterologist in Southern California, envisioned expanding his practice through the use of cutting-edge technology and service lines that he was uniquely qualified to provide through specialized training. His passion was embracing technologically advanced treatments in order to bring improved options to patients for optimum comfort and health while promoting education and healthy lifestyles in regard to his field.

Dr. Simoni's bedside manner and standard of care were impeccable, yet growth had been very slow in a competitive community landscape with long-established colleagues of the same specialty. In fact, although Dr. Simoni was the only specialist in the county who was trained in and offering a new and successful procedure known as transoral incisionless fundoplication (TIF) to treat the common ailment gastroesophageal reflux disease (GERD), he'd performed this procedure on only a few local patients at the time we first met with him. Though the procedure resulted in life-changing relief for patients, he was not attracting enough new interest.

We were called in to create a marketing plan for his practice, Advanced GI, Inc., and got to work immediately on demographic research, observing the practice, and completing a marketing SWOT analysis (examination of strengths, weaknesses, opportunities, and threats). This included patient interviews, mystery patient calls, and competitive analysis.

Our analysis revealed many opportunities, and among them was the need to rebrand this practice. Dr. Simoni understood the need for branding, and had already worked with a designer in creating a logo he believed summed up his practice perfectly. The problem was that Dr. Simoni himself had led the process and directed the designer in using digestive organs and an acronym for the practice logo. The result was a dark-colored, overly clinical, literal logo that didn't communicate the personality or desired image of the practice (Figure 1).

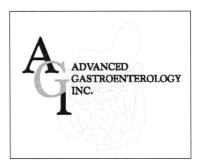

FIGURE 1. Sample of a "before" logo that is not patient-centered. Courtesy of Gilbert Simoni, MD.

The acronym (AGI) made identifying the practice difficult, giving it no memorable qualities and sounding more like an insurance company than a specialty medical practice. The ghost-imprint of intestines behind it was disturbing for those not used to working on the insides of people. To Dr. Simoni, these body parts represented years of study, a passion for his specialty, and his commitment to his patients. But branding must be palatable to your patients to maximize the benefit to your practice. Not only was the literal logo an outdated approach, but for patients who sometimes stress for days before a colonoscopy, seeing digestive organs on a business card is not a comfort and can be disturbing. All of this was a distraction from the innovative comfort and patient-centered care this practice aims to provide to each patient.

A logo is not a badge you wear but a mode of communication of all that you do and stand for *from your patients' perspective*. Clearly Dr. Simoni was bringing much more than "digestive organs" to his patients. His passion for preventative care, early detection of digestive diseases, and technologically advanced treatments to improve the quality of life for patients was being lost in his branding and marketing and therefore not communicated to the community or his referral sources.

His mission of bringing technologically advanced treatment and patient-friendly education to his patients was much broader than this logo communicated. Where were the "patient-friendly" and 'technologically advanced" elements in this logo? The logo was devoid of any of this meaning because it was so narrow and literal. Can you imagine the intestines on a t-shirt should the office staff participate in a future fundraising walk?

Dr. Simoni was eager to hear our point of view and respected our expertise. Although he was proud of the logo he had worked hard to create, he was also willing to consider how the logo might induce fear and discomfort in the minds of patients. We helped him realize that the existing logo was not a comfort to patients likely feeling apprehensive about their visits or procedures. And though it may be subliminal and patients may not even recognize it themselves, they really don't want to be forced to think about any intestines outside a body, but most importantly theirs!

After delving deeper to understand Dr. Simoni, his passion for innovation, his patient-friendly approach, and his vision for the practice, we were able to define his practice identity. We also worked with the practice to clarify its mission, and the following mission statement was created: "Our Mission is to build patient trust and to be the catalyst for a healthier lifestyle through prevention, early detection and our innovative approach to GI care." This statement helped lead the way in developing a clear identity and brand that patients could relate to and staff could embrace and deliver on.

A professional graphic designer was chosen who listened to Dr. Simoni's needs as well as our input as to what needed to be communicated to patients. With open communication and a few rounds of feedback and revision, branding was accomplished that the practice can grow with. It's simple, pleasant, memorable, and yet very professional—portraying the credible, patient-friendly, and innovative aspects of the practice.

A style board was created to help guide all future design work (Figure 2), from the Web site to ads and brochures. And a new logo (Figure 3) was designed that is fresh and modern, simple and clear. The colors used in the old logo were dark and serious; the new logo was designed using fresh, appealing colors and printed on bright white paper to evoke an overall clean, crisp, sophisticated yet friendly approach. The logo mark gives a nod to the digestive system without being overly literal, and the typography used in the practice name discretely conveys "high-tech," as does the practice name, which is now spelled out in the logo.

By defining the image of this practice in a fresh, patient-centered manner, consistent with Dr. Simoni's vision for Advanced GI's future and the practice's personality, we, in essence, revitalized the physician and staff as they felt prepared and hopeful that a well-thought-out *marketing plan* would showcase the practice in the community.

We could almost feel the increased energy and enthusiasm as we worked with Dr. Simoni on executing new marketing strategies and helping him build the practice he dreamed of—a practice that understood its strengths and was learning how to communicate and leverage them.

Dr. Simoni's practice personality, which is both forward-thinking and patient-centered, was now being communicated clearly and consistently through the practice Web site, brochures, business cards, and advertisements. This was the beginning of setting him up for the successful implementation of our marketing plan in a patient-centered

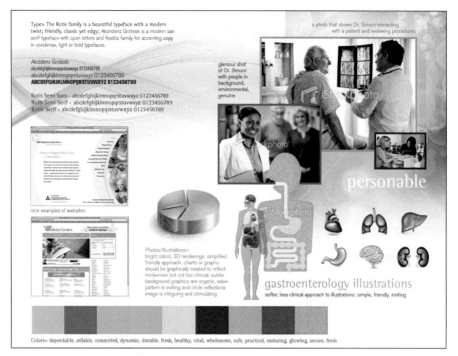

FIGURE 2. Sample of a style board, created by Kristin Borg Design Group, Inc., for Advanced GI, Inc. Used courtesy of Gilbert Simoni, MD.

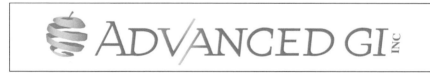

FIGURE 3. Sample of an "after" logo that illustrates a patient-centered approach to branding that communicates the identity of the practice. Created by Kristin Borg Design Group, Inc., and used courtesy of Gilbert Simoni, MD.

and consistent way that appealed to both referring physicians and potential patients in the community.

Advanced GI gained a great deal of traction over the next year. We reintroduced the practice to the community and potential referral sources with the practice's fresh look and appeal. We leveraged Dr. Simoni's personable style and ability to teach through public speaking, and we utilized the growing list of success stories from GERD sufferers who'd found life-changing relief through his offered procedure, thus creating visibility for the practice with its unique offering and experience in the TIF procedure.

Advanced GI's physician referral base expanded, and word of mouth resulted in more patient-directed referrals. Dr. Simoni soon gained the reputation of being the "go to" doctor for GERD sufferers in his community and was named one of the top providers of the procedure in the state and country. He sponsored community health events, had a patient's success story featured in the local newspaper, began partnering with the nonprofit Esophageal Cancer Action Network to raise awareness of the risks associated with GERD, and was asked to start training physicians from all over the country to perform the TIF procedure.

His desire to be a frontrunner in bringing advanced technology to his patients was finally giving him a competitive advantage in the community and setting him apart as a leader in his specialty. Did a new logo and mission statement create all this growth? It was the beginning of setting a new identity in motion, something the entire practice could begin to grow with. It influenced the culture of the practice and attitude of the physician to embrace the marketing plan and strategies with fervor and anticipation, which contributed to the success of their implementation.

GETTING IT RIGHT

Branding alone cannot bring success to a struggling practice, but defining your identity, crafting your mission, and creating your brand are the perfect starting places and are crucial to optimal success in competitive markets. Just like you wouldn't go to an important meeting or party in your workout or gardening clothes, you want to have your best "outfit" on before you begin to market your practice—something that truly represents the practice and elevates its strengths. Just as a wedding dress or tuxedo is altered in preparation for a wedding in order to fit exactly right, to accentuate the wearer's best features and conceal flaws, so it is with defining your mission and brand identity. Getting them right will feel good, give you confidence, and give your team something to get behind while emphasizing your strengths.

CONSISTENCY

Once your image is determined and guidelines are in place—such as font types, uniform colors, and specific messages in your Web site copy and collateral—consistency is essential. If you are attempting to portray a pampering spa-like environment to attract patients for cosmetic services, then untailored, mismatched scrubs are not a good choice for staff apparel. The specialist who touts his or her cutting-edge technology and embrace of the latest treatments has an inconsistent message when the reception room décor or Web site looks out of date and neglected. A strong, distinct image must be communicated repeatedly and consistently through marketing and brand development strategies that build patient confidence and industry credibility. Working with a healthcare marketer to develop your image and communicate it consistently will give your practice a strong, distinct image and recognition that when backed by action will attract and retain your desirable patients and ultimately position you for great success!

THE PAYOFF

Knowing who you are as a practice or other healthcare organization is essential to building a brand identity that differentiates you from the competition and attracts the patients you find most rewarding to serve. Professional guidance can lead to developing and leveraging a strong, patient-centered image in a market where success has become increasingly dependent on patient perception.

CHAPTER 4

The 24x7 Patient Relationship

CONTRIBUTING AUTHOR:
Laurie Morgan
Senior Consultant, Capko & Company

Do you think the Internet revolution has proceeded without you? Think again. Like the old saying about the ostrich burying its head in the sand, just because you can't see the people searching for you online doesn't mean they can't see you. Whether you help craft it or not, you've got an online reputation. The question is, will you take responsibility for how it helps—or hurts—your practice, or will you leave that up to chance?

J UST AS THE MANAGED CARE REVOLUTION has irrevocably altered the relationship between payers and physicians, the Internet revolution has done the same for patients' relationships with their healthcare providers. The explosion of online healthcare information sources has contributed to a more empowered and demanding patient population, and has completely changed the way patients find, choose, and interact with healthcare providers.

It all started innocently enough: publishers like WebMD and Yahoo! Health put information online in the late 1990s, and "Dr. Google" was born. Patients also began replacing their use of print yellow pages with online searches for local medical providers. Eventually, the Web 2.0 trend—the social use of the Web for consumer ratings, blogging, and eventually interacting through social networks like Facebook and Twitter—moved into healthcare.

Today, patients are not just researching physicians and healthcare organizations online, they're reading, evaluating, and even contributing to reviews and ratings of providers. They're gathering information about you and your practice even when your practice is closed. Even patients who've been referred to your practice by a friend or their primary care physician are going online before they come to see you—both to research their health problems and to learn more about you.

PATIENTS SEARCH FOR INFORMATION

You studied for years to become a physician—and continue to stay on top of your field by reading and analyzing stacks of medical literature. Now a patient comes in with a pile of articles printed from the Web, and she seems ready to second-guess whatever you have to say. Is the patient disrespectful of your credentials? Doesn't she trust you?

With research showing that 80% of people search for health information, including 66% seeking information about specific health problems,[1] chances are good that a significant proportion of your patients will arrive in your exam room armed with data from the Internet. The good news is, it's not about questioning your judgment; it's about engaging and taking responsibility for their role in maintaining their own health. The bad news is, misunderstanding patients' intentions can backfire.

> *Chances are good that a significant*
> *proportion of your patients will arrive*
> *in your exam room armed with data from*
> *the Internet.*

Today's patients are keenly aware that their time with you will be limited. They want to be prepared. Possibly, they're concerned or even quite afraid. If you or your staff members react to that preparation with frustration and an assumption of "cyberchondria," patients will feel disrespected and dismissed—and even though they may say nothing, they may already be planning to leave your practice before they've left the exam room. Worse, they may tell others how badly they were affected by the interaction with your practice. In the worst cases, if the assumption of cyberchondria causes providers or staff to discourage communication, patients may leave without getting the care they need.

Patients who do reams of research before their appointments may not realize that there won't be time during their visit to go through every article they found. Develop a strategy for gently managing their expectations—allowing you to make your diagnosis first, and answer a few specific questions afterwards. Help patients understand how to identify the few sites they should be looking at for credible information. Helping *all* of your patients understand which Web sites offer credible information and support and which don't is a great marketing opportunity for your practice—and a great way to minimize the amount of debunking of bad information you'll have to do during visits.

DIRECTORIES RULE PHYSICIAN SEARCHES

Of course, all that health-related Web searching patients are doing includes the search for a doctor. When they're looking for a new provider, are you showing up in their path?

Do a search on any specialty in any city, and the top 10 results will almost always include numerous directory listings: Google Places, physician rating sites, hospital directories, yellow pages sites, and health plan directories. It's not uncommon for directory listings to show up first *even for searches on your name*—especially if you have no Web site or if your Web site is not well optimized for search. It's essential to ensure that you are listed correctly in these directories.

There are a shocking number of ways in which your directory information can be incorrect. Have you moved recently? Some sites are probably relying on outdated information, and so list you at your former address or practice. (Imagine how a patient will react to showing up at the wrong place for his appointment. Hurried patients looking up your address and directions on their smartphones on the way to their visit can have this exact experience if the first listing that pops up for your name is outdated.)

Did you recently graduate? Some directories may not list you at all. Do you have a common name? Some directories may have your identity completely confused—or fused—with that of another physician. If you practice in a subspecialty, that information will likely be missing from directory sites. If you've added or deleted health plans, it's also quite likely that those directories are not accurate, and you may be losing prospective patients as a result.

Maintaining accurate directory listings should be the responsibility of directory publishers, but they unfortunately make frequent mistakes that inconvenience patients and can reflect badly on your practice. By taking responsibility for verifying and updating this information, you'll help protect your patient service reputation and ease the path for new patients to find you.

START WITH HEALTH PLAN DIRECTORIES

Inaccurate information in payer directories can wreak silent havoc with your patient marketing efforts. Most patients will want to confirm that your practice accepts their insurance before contacting you. If you're not listed in a directory for a plan you accept, you are in effect turning prequalified prospective patients away. Being incorrectly listed as "not accepting new patients" has the same effect.

But as bad as being incorrectly excluded from a payer directory is, being incorrectly *included* in the directories of plans you've dropped has the potential to cause much bigger problems. What if a referred patient schedules a visit, only to find out afterwards that she has been seen out-of-network—and now there's a significant balance to pay? Your practice will be paid less than it should be by the payer, the patient will be stuck with a large unexpected bill (which you may end up writing off), and more likely than not, the patient's bad experience will be shared with friends, coworkers, relatives, and possibly the entire Internet via a ratings site.

Inaccuracies in payer directory listings are not rare. In fact, they're so common (and problematic to consumers) that the state attorney general in New York recently sued a group of health plans to force them to commit to better maintenance of their directories.[2] It would be nice if your practice could rely on payers to tighten up their editing procedures in your market, but the accuracy of this information is too vital to your practice to leave up to someone else. Practice staff members need to set reminders to check this information every few months. And when signing up with a new plan, make a point of staying in touch with the plan to confirm your information is properly added as quickly as possible.

GRAB YOUR GOOGLE PLACES LISTING

If you've searched on a local business recently, you may have noticed that a group of listings keyed to a map appears near the top of the page, as you can see from this search for "plumber san francisco" shown in Figure 1.

The listings starting with ogradyplumbing.com match the locations pinned on the map at the upper right—and highlight that the listings come with reviews. Now if you mouse over ogradyplumbing.com's listing (just to the right of the address), up pops an expanded listing with an image (Figure 2).

Interestingly, every plumber listed has at least one photo. If you were to do a similar search on a medical specialty, you'd also see a

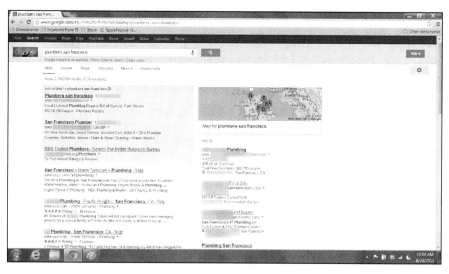

FIGURE 1.

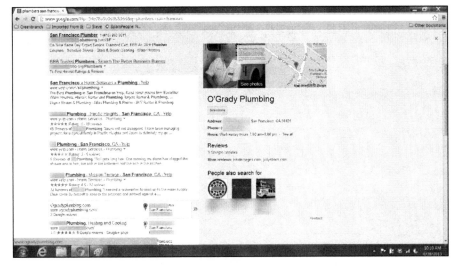

FIGURE 2.

group of Google Places listings, but almost none would be custom-ized with photos and descriptive information—even here in "wired" San Francisco! Physician practices have been slow to embrace the marketing potential of Google's listings. This presents a great oppor-tunity for those practices that do claim and customize their listings to really stand out from the pack, and it costs nothing except a bit of your time.

> *It is best to start with one social*
> *network first, and focus on building*
> *an audience and serving it effectively*
> *before adding another.*

Even if you haven't claimed your listing, you may already have a skeletal one that Google assembled based on other information online about you: your name, location (possibly inaccurate, if Google relied on outdated sources), and phone number such as the example shown in Figure 3.

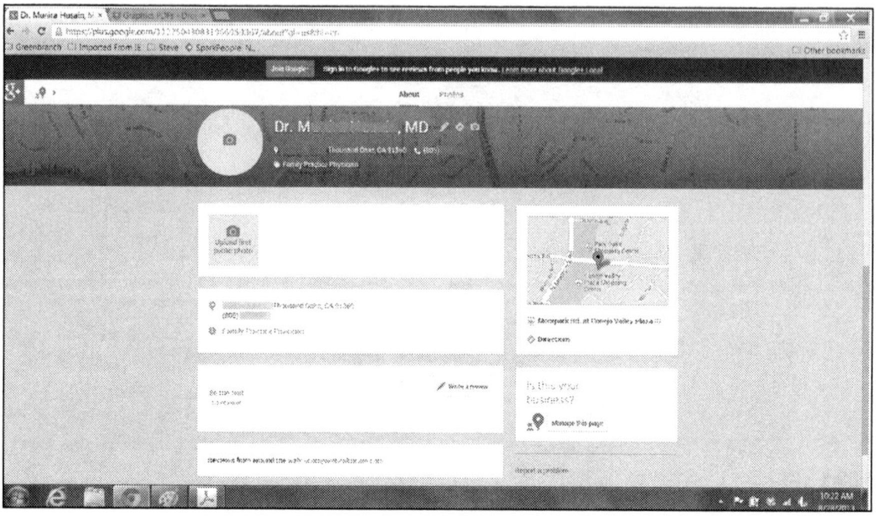

FIGURE 3.

Notice the grey button that says "Manage this page" in the right hand column of the page. Clicking on this allows you to enter or update your listing (including embellishing it with photos, your office hours, and your own description).

Once you've completed your changes, Google will need to verify your ownership of the listing before publishing it (to prevent unauthorized people from changing your profile); this is done by delivering a PIN to your office either through an automated call to your published phone number (not feasible if no employee answers the phone directly) or via a mailing (usually an easier option for practices) (Figure 4).

If you don't see even a skeletal listing, you can create your own entirely from scratch by setting up a Google account (just visit www. google.com/places).

Google listings are so likely to pop up near the top in any Web search for you or your specialty, it's essential to claim them and make sure they're providing your patients with accurate information.

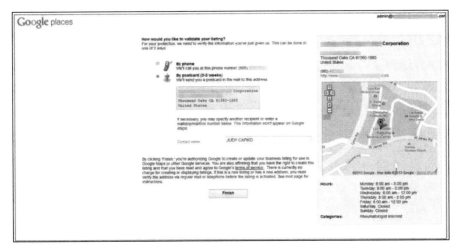

FIGURE 4.

DON'T RUN FROM RATINGS AND REVIEWS

You may have noticed that the Google listings include reviews—not just from their own visitors, but also sometimes from other sites, most commonly Vitals.com, Healthgrades.com, or local interest sites (e.g., parenting-oriented sites for pediatricians). Naturally, these reviews are not always 100% positive—and that can cause some consternation. But don't let the presence of reviews—even negative ones—discourage you from actively managing the other content of these listings. There are powerful reasons to deal with these listings to the extent you can, even when you feel that a site has permitted patients to paint an unfair picture of you and your practice.

One important reason: negative review content sometimes contains valuable feedback that you need to hear—and you might not hear it through any other source. It's often the case that negative reviews are related to the nonclinical side of the patient experience: the appointment-setting process, staff friendliness, comfort of the waiting area, and billing and collections. It's unfortunate when these

45

activities reflect poorly on you, but *learning that patients are dissatisfied with these aspects of your practice is a gift*. These are the exact kinds of problems that can lead patients to quietly leave your practice without telling you why. Reading online reviews can open your eyes to hidden problems that are within your control to fix.

Of course, you might encounter a review that you believe is unduly negative or unrealistically presents the constraints of patient care. It's not usually possible to persuade a review site to remove a review unless it's clearly irrelevant or dishonest (e.g., obviously written by someone who was not your patient). (Google and Yelp, for example, both offer the opportunity to flag as inappropriate any review that appears to violate these guidelines.) Some sites allow the option to publicly respond to reviews; while privacy concerns are paramount and will limit what you're able to add to a public site, you can at least demonstrate your interest in patient service by encouraging posters to contact your office to discuss concerns privately and in person. Some sites permit a private response—better still for sensitive issues. But even in those cases, the private response medium is best used to encourage the poster to connect with you offline for further discussion.

> ### Negative reviews probably contain valuable feedback that you, as a practice executive, need to hear.

It's important to remember that a small proportion of negative reviews is unlikely to drive patients away from your practice, especially when the gripes are unrelated to patient care. Most patients understand that "nobody's perfect," and may even take a few negatives mixed in with positive reviews as a sign that the process is credible (and not biased by reviews from a few close fans of your practice). Try to learn from the negative feedback to improve your practice, but also try not to get overly exercised about it.

Taking an active role in managing your online listings is a natural step toward engaging your patients more with your practice and actively seeking their feedback while they're at your practice. Some of the more prominent ratings and reviews sites, such as Vitals.com and Yelp.com, provide local businesses with materials to help them encourage patients to contribute reviews. The best way to counteract a negative review or two is to encourage more satisfied patients to contribute their views, especially if you've taken steps to address valid feedback.

Patient satisfaction is becoming an important quality metric to payers. Developing your practice's own processes for understanding how your patients experience it can help you get ahead of the trend. It shows your patients that you are interested in their concerns, and that sends the message that you care. You may even find that gathering your own feedback from patients has a side effect of better ratings on public sites, because many people feel better about a service experience just as a result of being asked for feedback (and so may be less inclined to go online to complain).

CLAIMING YOUR LISTINGS ON RATINGS SITES

The number of review and rating sites for healthcare organizations continues to grow. (This is yet another reason to monitor these sites and work with them to keep your published details accurate; they're not going away any time soon.) In addition to a growing number of places where all physician specialties can be listed and reviewed, there are specialty-specific sites emerging, such as RealSelf.com for plastic surgery and ObesityHelp.com for bariatric medicine and surgery.

As of this writing, though, two sites still stand out as the most consequential for the majority of practices because they're consistently at the top of the results for searches: Vitals.com and Healthgrades.

com. Claiming your listings on these sites and verifying and updating them should be your first priority because these listings reach huge numbers of people in search results.

To claim your listings on these sites, you'll need identifying information like your state license number and/or NPI number (for yourself and/or your practice). The sites use this information (along with a postal mailing in the case of Vitals.com) to confirm your identity and block unauthorized editing of profiles.

Once you've verified and updated your information on Google Places, Vitals.com, and Healthgrades.com, you can begin working through other places where you're listed to ensure their accuracy and monitor any posted reviews. The book *Establishing, Managing, and Protecting Your Online Reputation* (Greenbranch Publishing, 2013) by Dr. Kevin Pho ("KevinMD.com") and Susan Gay has a helpful list of secondary rating sites to help you get started.

AUTOMATED EAVESDROPPING

Setting up accounts and claiming listings on directories can be a first step toward monitoring what patients are saying about you and your practice, since some of these sites notify registered physicians and administrators when new reviews or ratings are added to their listings.

But with new sites popping up every day, and physician ratings also being added to nonmedical sites, it's useful to cast a broader net. Most of us don't have time to Google ourselves every day to see if anything new appears, even though that would be ideal. Thankfully, Google has simplified the process of keeping tabs on what's being said online through its Google Alerts service (google.com/alerts).

This service permits you to set up any number of e-mail alerts to monitor whatever keywords you choose, and it's free. You can use it to monitor what's being said about you and your practice, as well as other topics of interest. For example, if you're interested in the direct-pay practice model or what's happening with a particular local employer or health plan, you can set up alerts for appropriate keywords to hear about new information on the subject as soon as it hits the Web.

Finding out what's happening on blogs and Web sites of interest to you is a great way to identify online conversations that you'll want to jump into, which, in turn, is a great way to bolster your visibility and positively influence your reputation. If you are able to provide a link back to your own Web site with your comments, you'll give your own site a boost—helping to improve the likelihood that it's the first result returned when people search locally on your name or specialty.

YES, YOU NEED A WEB SITE

With so many places a practice can be listed online today, it may seem that your practice can do without a Web site of its own. But having your own home online—a place where you have total control over how you're presented—is a powerful tool in establishing your online personality. What's more, it provides a platform for you to share information with large numbers of patients at once—showing how much you care, and doing it efficiently.

Of course, to leverage the power of a practice Web site to connect with patients, you need to have a Web site that is easily updated by you or your staff. If you're stuck with an older Web site that can be modified only by a developer, you're sacrificing your site's potential to help you connect with patients on your own timetable. And you're likely over-paying for those updates. A modern Web site, created in a content management system such as WordPress, is one of the highest return-on-investment marketing and communication investments you can make for your practice. Sites created in WordPress are easy to modify and update—the WordPress platform originated as a blogging tool, designed to enable anyone to easily publish online. The current version offers more bells and whistles, but hasn't lost the simplicity that enables anyone to use it with minimal training.

A skilled WordPress developer can create a customized look and feel for your practice Web site with just a few weeks' work, usually for less than $5000. Developers can build off readily available starter templates that enable your site to be "responsive" (i.e., automatically adjusting for smartphone and tablet screen sizes) so that patients can easily access your site from whatever device they're using. Make sure the design reflects your practice's personality and integrates with the look and feel of any other marketing materials you're using (logo, brochures, signs, business cards).

A modern Web site is one of the highest return-on-investment expenditures you can make for your practice.

Including a blog with your site will enable you to publish your own articles and announcements easily—for example, you can share links to news stories about health studies that you find credible (with comments on how patients might use the information). When studies that create a lot of controversy hit the headlines—say, unusual dietary research or modified screening guidelines—posting your view on your Web site can save your practice a lot of time if it cuts down on phone calls to staff. And, of course, it's a lot easier for your patients, too! If your patients find an article link they appreciate on your Web site, they may share it on social media—another form of passive marketing that can help enhance your practice's reputation. (Make sure your site has sharing buttons in place to make this easier.)

Publishing new information on your Web site—whether via a blog you add to regularly or just by updating your home page with news and information—is one of the best ways to improve your site's visibility in search results, known as search engine optimization (SEO). Effective SEO, in turn, helps increase the likelihood that your own site will be found near the top of a search for you or your specialty so that you get the chance to virtually "speak" to prospective and current patients who look for you online, and are less at the mercy of how other information sources present your practice. Even if you don't have the time to post daily, or even weekly, a little bit of new content every month or so goes a long way toward reminding Google and the other search engines that your site exists and is being maintained. This is their signal that the same is true of your practice.

ADDING MORE VALUE TO YOUR SITE

The ability to add relevant content as needed is one of the best ways your site can add value for patients. A few other really simple ways to increase your site's usefulness for patients are to add Google maps (for directions to your office) and an updated calendar/office hours (another great reason to have a site you can update yourself so you can change this information in response to holidays, bad weather, etc).

Adding downloadable new-patient forms—easy to set-up and update with a content management system—is another way to make things easier for both your patients and your staff.

Enabling patients to access their health information online is a more substantial project. Adding a portal link to your Web site is easy, but selecting the right portal and integrating it effectively and securely with your electronic medical record and practice management systems are more technical, complex, and demanding projects. But embarking on them also has the potential for a much larger payoff in patient satisfaction and practice efficiency.

As more and more people become accustomed to 24x7 self-management of all kinds of critical personal information online—banking, credit cards, taxes—it's natural to see why many observers expect access to electronic health records via patient portals to be a huge step forward in patient service. It also has the potential to enable your practice to run more efficiently, by allowing patients to submit requests via secure electronic communication, receive lab results and request prescription renewals without a phone call, and book appointments themselves online. A portal is also the most direct path to meeting many "Meaningful Use" measures, such as delivering electronic copies of medical records within three business days of the patient's request, delivering patient-specific education materials, providing patients with a clinical summary of their visit, and providing timely notifications to patients about changes to their health records.

GOING SOCIAL

"Social media." It's a phrase that still seems to make physicians and practice managers a bit nervous, especially considering the challenges it seems to present in maintaining patient privacy and meeting patient expectations for responsiveness. Yet with so many patients now using social platforms like Facebook, Twitter, and, increasingly, Google+, it also seems clear that social media could offer valuable opportunities to engage patients and reach them more efficiently. What is the right way to proceed for your practice?

The answer is not one-size-fits-all for every practice, and the question really prompts more questions. Fortunately, it's not necessary to take part in all of the social media possibilities to gain some of the benefits of participating. For example, simply visiting other people's blogs and commenting on them and making your own Web site content easily shareable on social networks are low-investment ways to participate in community connections while remaining mostly on the sidelines.

If you're seriously considering adding a Facebook or Google+ presence or starting a Twitter feed to help promote your practice and engage patients, it's critical to think through your goals for doing so. Social networks are intolerant of anything that looks like pure promotion; sharing via social networks must have perceived value to the community. Maintaining a social media presence can also entail a fair amount of work because there are high expectations for fast responses to questions, messages, and comments. Physicians also have to be vigilant about ensuring that privacy is protected when patients interact with them on social sites.

Start by being a social media user.
Join groups that follow subjects that matter
to you and your comfort level will grow.

Because of the added workload, it is best to start with one social network first, and focus on building an audience and serving it effectively before adding another. Keep in mind also that it may not be worth the investment of time and energy if your practice specialty is not one that naturally fosters patient communities. For example, a Facebook page might be a natural fit for an OB/GYN or pediatric practice, since patients enjoy sharing experiences and hearing ongoing tips and ideas from their providers. But many radiologists or surgical specialists may find less potential benefit to their patients or their practices from attempting to create a community online.

Connecting with patients via social media requires special care to separate your practice identity from your personal one. Facebook introduced the concept of "business pages" that allow organizations to engage with their customers at a bit of a distance compared with the "friend" model of personal Facebook accounts, and Google+ has followed suit. On Twitter, it's possible to set up as many accounts with different handles as you like (at least as many as you have e-mail addresses).

Perhaps the best way to understand the expectations patients will have from your social media interactions—as well as the possibilities for your practice—is to first experience social media yourself as a *user*. Sign up for your own Facebook and/or Google+ account, reconnect with friends (real friends—not patients!), join groups that follow subjects that matter to you, and like pages for brands, publications, and organizations you appreciate. This way, when you're ready to create a social media identity for your practice, you'll already have an understanding of how the network you choose works for users, and an appreciation for potential pitfalls.

Is someone on your staff a social media maven? Perhaps you can tap his or her skills and create a social media team for your practice. Provided that you've worked out a strategy for dealing with patient over-sharing of personal information ("Thank you for posting, Ms. Jones, please call us so that we can discuss your concerns privately.") or who have negative feedback ("We're sorry to hear that your expectations weren't met. Would you be willing to contact us offline so that we can understand what happened?"), it's possible to empower several people to monitor a practice's social media identify. This helps ensure patients' high expectations for response time are met. Remember, though, to monitor who has access and delete administrative privileges when staff members leave your practice, to avoid sabotage or neglect of your social media identity.

EMBRACING COMMUNITY

One of the main appeals of social media is the easy means it offers for people to congregate and to form and extend relationships. People who didn't know each other offline—who perhaps live in different parts of the country—might find they can help each other cope with a health problem by joining the same group for people with their illness.

In many ways, social media replaces community gatherings that used to happen more commonly in the offline world. If you're leery of the 24x7 nature of a social media presence but still interested in engaging patients more fully with your practice, the "old school" approach can be a great alternative. Open houses, wellness lectures, Saturday flu shot clinics, and group visits are all ways to connect with patients beyond the office visit and demonstrate your practice's concern for their well-being.

Developing an e-mail list of your patients enables you to promote events like these and stay connected in other ways, too—for example, your practice could create a quarterly newsletter. Use your patient information forms to collect e-mail addresses from patients, and be sure there's a space to indicate whether they've agreed to receive nonclinical information ("opted in").

LAST BUT NOT LEAST: PROFESSIONAL SOCIAL MEDIA

Social networking with professional colleagues on career-oriented networks gets less attention, but using these networks can be easier to manage and indirectly help your practice become more patient-centered.

Sermo, for example, is a network that is 100% restricted to physicians, who can post to discussions anonymously—a safe environment for sharing ideas and problems with peers. As being more patient-focused and measuring service quality become more important to physicians, there will undoubtedly be benefit to exchanging questions, experiences, and ideas on this subject with like-minded physicians.

LinkedIn, the business social network, is often ignored by physicians and practice staff, but it is easy to use and has helpful reputation effects. Your LinkedIn profile includes space for your Web site link, which means it contributes to SEO for your site; and it is often the case that a search on a doctor who is on LinkedIn will show his or her LinkedIn profile as the first result. (This is much preferable to a directory listing showing up in that spot, since a person has complete control over his or her LinkedIn profile.) You may also set up a company page for your practice on LinkedIn. While LinkedIn is unlikely to be the first place patients will turn for practice information, it's a helpful tool, and it offers easy control over content. Once signed up, there are also opportunities to join many professional groups that offer useful networking discussions about business and professional issues.

THE PAYOFF

The explosion of online healthcare information is contributing to a more empowered patient population. It has changed the way patients find, choose, and interact with healthcare providers. By taking the initiative with online media, healthcare providers and organizations can manage their online reputations, increase patient engagement, and boost marketing efforts to attract potential new patients.

References

1. Fox S. The Social Life of Health Information. Pew Internet Research. May 2011; www.pewinternet.org/Reports/2011/Social-Life-of-Health-Info.aspx.
2. A.G. Schneiderman Announces Settlements Requiring Health Insurers To Publish Accurate Provider Directories. New York State Office of the Attorney General. January 19, 2012; www.ag.ny.gov/press-release/ag-schneiderman-announces-settlements-requiring-health-insurers-publish-accurate.

CHAPTER 5

What's Wrong with This Picture?

Most physicians know who they are—what makes them tick and how they intend to distinguish themselves from their competitors—and the image they want for their practice. But a clear public portrayal of that image isn't everything. The most well-written mission statement, a patient-friendly logo, and a beautifully scripted Web site do not ensure that the practice makes good on these implied promises. Although the image your practice portrays is vitally important, the culture inside your practice has the greatest impact on the patient experience. When the image and patient experience are not in sync, patients are confused and disenchanted; they know there is something very wrong with this picture.

SO YOU KNOW YOUR MISSION, and you are ready to conquer the world—or at least your little corner of it—by being the *best*, with quality care and stellar *customer service*. You get the staff on board, and everyone's pumped up to deliver. You start out strong, but somewhere down the line everyone seems to run out of steam. Staff members fall back into old habits of displaying less-than-enthusiastic attitudes, and pushing patients through the system until 5:00 PM seems to be the only goal on anyone's mind. You know patients aren't impressed; no one is. Yet someone started this quest, and everyone was on board at the time. What went wrong?

LIVING THE MISSION

Often the best intentions are not lived out in the actions necessary to succeed. It's an old adage, but actions *do* speak louder than words, especially for patients. Defining your practice mission doesn't change the practice culture (though it's a fantastic place to start). Breaking down how you will live out the mission doesn't change the practice culture—even though it's an essential step in living up to it. Only a change of actions and attitudes will truly impact the practice culture. Defining your mission and how it will be attained are important beginning steps, but then comes the commitment to actually *do* it.

As leaders of a practice, hospital, or other medical facility, the administrators, managers, and physicians hold the place of greatest cultural influence because they set the tone and also set the bar. No, everyone won't always follow suit, we know that all too well—but when leaders are in sync with their mission and display the core values of an organization from within, the impact is so great, so powerful, and so valuable that it's almost impossible *not* to succeed. Couple this with accountability and performance measurements that provide leaders with the ability to weed out or provide additional

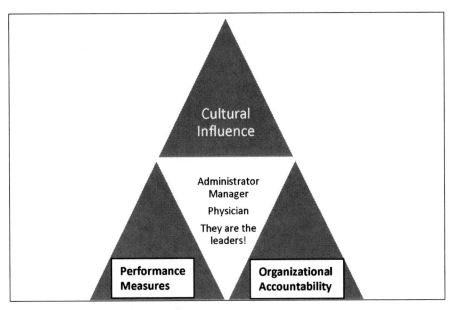

FIGURE 1. Cultural influence.

training to those who are not meeting the mark, and you have put yourself in the league of best practices (Figure 1).

IT'S TIME FOR A REALITY CHECK

The case studies in this chapter will reveal the types of costly mistakes a hospital or medical practice can make when it is inconsistent in its message and actions or fails to follow through on its promises or commitment to being patient-centered. This often results in confusing patients, compromising customer service, and contributing to a high attrition rate. It is actually a form of de-marketing and can be very destructive to the image and reputation of a medical practice, Accountable Care Organization, hospital, or healthcare system.

These case studies will help you understand the importance of knowing why you exist and making it the primary focus of what you do and how you deliver your services. By reading these stories, you will likely realize how easy it is to get wrapped up in the processes and the technical part of getting patients through the system rather than focusing on each patient as an individual that is vulnerable and has needs. You and your staff can meet these needs by first being more aware of them, then striving to achieve patient service goals that result in a commitment to improve consistency between the message you portray to the public and patients' perceptions of your practice, and finally by delivering a stellar customer service experience. It takes the commitment of everyone in the practice to consistently meet the expectations of patients. It is essential to being a patient-centered practice.

CASE STUDY

Image Collision

Jonathan Weston, MD, is a partner with City Center Cardiology and Chief of Cardiology at the most reputable hospital in town. The practice has been investing in advertising for some time, touting Dr. Weston's incredible expertise and special training. The practice logo, Web site, and marketing collateral are impressive, complementing the practice's brand and image. Dr. Weston is active in the community and a seasoned public speaker. He has given a number of presentations, sharing his expertise with other physicians and the community at large, which has increased the flow of new patients into City Center Cardiology. Unfortunately, the impressive image ends when the patient arrives at the practice, just ask Mary Shock.

Mary Shock was home alone, her three children were at school, and her husband was on a business trip. She felt a funny sensation and a fluttering in her chest; it wasn't the first time. She tried to ignore it, but it seemed to get worse and concerned her enough to call her primary care practice where she was seen later that day. After running a few tests, her physician felt that although there was nothing to be alarmed about, Mary should have a cardiac workup. She recommended Dr. Weston and told Mary he was the Chief of Cardiology at her hospital of choice, which was well known for its Heart Institute. Mary knew about Dr. Weston; she heard him speak at the hospital, saw some of the ads City Center Cardiology ran in local publications, and even saw a human interest story with pictures of Dr. Weston and one of his patients. She frequently saw the practice's beautiful building with its great signage while driving on the expressway downtown. After being referred by her primary care physician, Mary checked out City Center Cardiology's Web site, and felt confident she would get the best cardiology care available in her community.

Mary called immediately to schedule an appointment, but when the receptionist answered with a mumbled voice, she wasn't sure she had the right office. She asked for clarification, and the receptionist unenthusiastically confirmed she'd reached City Center Cardiology, but then Mary found herself on hold. Eventually she was given an appointment a week later. When Mary arrived for her appointment, she expected to see a polished, contemporary reception room with ample space. Instead, the décor was unimpressive, in fact nothing matched—the flooring and wall colors weren't even coordinated. Everything clashed, including chrome-framed seating, traditional end tables, and baroque-framed Italian prints on the wall. A big-screen television was blasting away in a room too small to accommodate a group practice this size.

Mary walked up to the open window to discover a receptionist on the telephone. Without making eye contact and without a word to Mary, the receptionist pointed to a sign-in sheet and turned away from Mary to continue her conversation. Because she had a few questions, Mary waited for someone to help her rather than take a seat. Another receptionist appeared on the scene, but ignored her. Mary looked around as she waited. She noticed the reception window was covered with notices to patients on unframed paper, curling on the ends and taped all over the place. There were stacks of papers and files in the reception office—it was in total disarray. This did not look like the practice she had envisioned. From that point on, things just got worse.

Finally, when the first receptionist hung up the phone, she turned to Mary, looked at the sign-in sheet to see who she was, and then asked for her insurance card and *told* her to fill out a patient information form. There was no, "Welcome to our practice, how may I help you?"

There wasn't even a smile. It seemed cold and perfunctory, and Mary began to feel insignificant. She was told to take a seat in the waiting room and became a little perturbed.

She sat in one of the few unoccupied chairs and soon found out why they called it a *waiting room* instead of a reception room. It was 30 minutes later when someone called for Mary and led her to the exam room—walking at least 10 feet ahead of her. Mary assumed it was a nurse, but couldn't be sure since the person didn't introduce herself and wasn't wearing a badge or name tag. They stopped in the hallway for Mary to get on the scale, where there was no place to put her jacket or purse during the process. She felt uncomfortable and annoyed that she was being weighed where other people were walking by. She was then taken to an exam room where her name was written in dry erase marker on a plaque on the outside of the door. Inside, she found the room to be stark and the exam table uncomfortable, and she began to shiver as she waited in the crunchy paper gown. Mary began feeling some anxiety and wished she had thought to bring something to read. The wait seemed endless, as she listened to staff scurrying about outside her door; chatting and laughing within earshot of the exam room. She even heard someone talking to a patient about things she felt uncomfortable overhearing.

When Dr. Weston arrived, he was pleasant and mildly attentive. He had a wonderful, relaxed manner and took his time. He explained everything; and before he left the room, he told her his nurse would give her instructions and to just step out of the room when she was dressed and ready. At last Mary felt really cared for and understood why Dr. Weston enjoyed such a favorable reputation. She felt good. Then the nurse called her to a counter in the hallway and began discussing the studies that were ordered and explained how to prepare for these tests. She also had Mary sign consent forms. This was done without regard for privacy, as patients, staff, and other physicians walked back and forth. This was terribly uncomfortable for Mary, but when she mentioned it, the nurse quickly dismissed it. Once again, she felt discounted and unimportant.

By the time her visit was over, Mary wondered how in the world a practice that gives the patient this kind of experience can expect patients to be satisfied. Even if every physician in this practice has great clinical skills and bedside manners, she thought, what happened before and after her time in the exam room had ruined her experience. She would never refer a friend or family member to City Center Cardiology.

Mary recalled a visit to the local grocery store the day before that could have taught this practice something about customer service. She remembered how when she appeared puzzled while viewing items on a grocery shelf, an employee stopped and asked if she could be of help; and how when she waited in a line with four people ahead of her, another checker was called to assist with customers. The store seemed to care, she thought, so why doesn't this doctor's office care more? After all, the doctors are seeing sick and frightened patients. By the end of the day, Mary vowed never to return to City Center Cardiology. This practice did not live up to its perceived image and apparently wasn't concerned about providing good service.

We were called into this practice when its efforts to be visible in the community and secure its reputation were met with disappointing results and patient growth that was minimal. We took a serious look at the practice including onsite observations. To complete our analysis, we interviewed physicians, staff members, and patients, including Mary Shock. Our role was to provide an objective analysis and offer the practice recommendations that would result in making meaningful changes to improve patient service and achieve growth.

Analysis

1. An inconsistency existed between the desired image and what patients' actually experienced during visits. Though Dr. Weston provided excellent clinical care and had a fine bedside manner, the staff and protocol of the office did not put patients' needs first.
2. No objective *tangible* service performance metrics were established to hold staff accountable to a defined standard.
3. New staff orientation training was inconsistent with little attention to customer service.

4. Patient satisfaction surveys were nonexistent.

5. Patient satisfaction was not a performance measure used in conducting annual staff performance reviews and establishing employee compensation gains.

6. Front office staff did not have sufficient guidance and super-vision.

City Center Cardiology had great intentions and invested in efforts to create visibility for its physicians and showcase their skills. Unfortunately, its focus was primarily on interactions and activities outside the walls of the practice. The practice made a common mis-take by not analyzing the patient experience to identify what might need to change before it engaged in outreach and marketing the practice. When a practice fails to address its internal workings and the patient service it is providing, it risks the possibility that external marketing activities will result in a turnstile of new patients that are not impressed or sufficiently engaged with the patient experience to return for additional care. In addition, these non-returning patients can actually harm the practice's reputation by negative word-of-mouth discussions they are likely to have with their friends, family, and coworkers.

Recommendations

1. Conduct a baseline patient satisfaction survey to gather quan-titative information on where improvements could be made.

2. Engage a consultant to conduct a small sampling of patient post-encounter interviews to allow for dialogue, collecting qualitative information in order to gain a deeper understanding of patient needs and expectations.

3. Based on findings, conduct a physician and staff patient-service workshop and establish improvement goals.

4. Remeasure results in six months and quarterly thereafter.

5. Recruit and hire a front office supervisor.

Outcome

We prepared a marketing plan, including a SWOT (strengths, weak-nesses, opportunities, and threats) analysis, and worked closely with the practice for more than a year. We focused on overcoming its weaknesses and building on its strengths. We worked diligently with staff and management to develop a shared vision that supported the practice's mission. We involved everyone in the process, developing cross-department teams that helped unite management with staff, giving the staff a sense of pride and enhancing teamwork.

We helped recruit and hire a front office supervisor, Jenna Salazar, who had years of experience managing a solo-physician plastic surgery practice. She is masterful at delivering great customer service and a natural leader who inspired staff to share her zeal for putting patients first. She demonstrates to staff what she expects of them when interacting with patients by setting service standards and guiding staff to meet those standards. Her leadership and example, along with new measurement tools and staff training, had a dramatic impact on the culture of the practice and the experience of the patients. Six months after Jenna was hired, a patient satisfaction survey was performed, and the practice received stellar marks.

Warm smiles, eye contact, and introductions by staff became second nature. The new supervisor was able to improve the scheduling process and reduce wait times as well. Staff members who had been too busy to care before, now felt important and knew their contribution was valued. Patient satisfaction surveys were now a valued measurement and guided changes in response to patient needs. The front office staff members realized a new level of satisfaction in their own roles. A patient testimonial page was added to the practice's Web site, where glowing comments by patients were added, and the practice gained a stronger online reputation as patients rated it highly on review sites, thus leading to increased growth.

CASE STUDY

Off the Mark with Hospital Patient Service

This experience was quite personal for me (JC), as it involved my mother. At the age of 91, my mother was accidently knocked down on the sidewalk by a bicycle ridden by a child. An ambulance was summoned, and she was taken to the hospital of her choice. The last time she had been in a hospital was 45 years earlier when she lived in a different state, so she picked the relatively new hospital that was making a big splash in town with a massive campaign of advertising and community outreach.

I flew into town and went directly to the hospital. It was in a beautiful part of town, and the décor was lovely and spotless. I noticed an easel in the main lobby with a slick poster announcing its Pampered Guest Program, which boasted of the hospital's commitment to listen to patients and provide outstanding service. I was sure the typical visitor would be duly impressed.

Fortunately, Mom had only a hairline fracture of the pelvis, and she was waiting to be transported to the skilled nursing floor when I arrived. She seemed comfortable, but anxious to be moved. When she was finally moved around 1:00 PM, I noticed another Pampered Guest easel prominently placed in the hallway as we exited the elevator.

When we arrived at Mom's hospital room I was struck by the incredible panoramic view from the window. Wow—this would be the view my mother would wake up to and enjoy before turning out the lights at night. If this was any indication of the care she was going to receive, I knew she would be very pleased. Within a few minutes, a nurse came in to check on Mom and do all the clinical things needed to properly check her in. A hep lock was left in her arm when the IV was removed in the emergency department, and it was hurting her, so I asked the nurse if she could remove it. She rudely replied, "I can't do that, she needs a doctor's orders." I asked how we might go about getting that, and she barked, "I don't know, but the hospital doctor will *probably* come by before the end of the evening." I was floored by her attitude. This sure didn't seem like the Pampered Guest service the hospital was touting.

After I managed to get this problem solved, I asked the certified nursing assistant if we could get something for Mom to eat. Except for applesauce, Jell-O, and crackers, my mother had had nothing to eat since being admitted the evening before. The assistant was pleasant and accommodating. It took a while, but finally a tray was brought to my mother. Later on, a woman came by from the dietary services department. She introduced herself and gave my mother a menu to make her choices for dinner and the following day's meals. She asked if Mom had any special dietary requests, and said that if Mom wanted anything special to eat she could write it down on the menu, and her order would be picked up shortly. She also invited my mother to call between meals if she wanted a snack or any special food item. My mother was impressed, and so was I. After all, elderly people can be picky about what they eat and can have difficulty digesting some foods; and when they are sick, these issues can be magnified. It felt good to know the hospital was concerned enough to pay special attention to the food desires of its patients. We soon discovered that this may have been the hospital's intentions, but it simply could not deliver on this intention. My mother's meals were consistently delivered with foods other than what she ordered, and something as simple as a request for a liquid dietary supplement was seldom met.

On the second day of Mom's hospital stay, a social worker stopped in to interview her while I happened to be visiting. She introduced herself, gave each of us her business card, and communicated what her role would be in assisting my mother and explained what my mother could expect during her rehabilitation. The social worker asked how my mother's health, well-being, and safety would be managed when Mom returned home. She was thoughtfully concerned; however, her conversation was peppered with comments about how busy she was and how understaffed her department was. In fact, the social worker didn't have her own computer, so, she apologetically explained, there might be a delay in taking care of some details. This proved to be the case. I couldn't help but wonder how a hospital that couldn't meet the needs of its own employees expected to deliver on a promise to pamper its patients.

The next afternoon, a Pampered Guest representative stopped by to visit my mother, brought her the gift of a pen and note cards, and inquired about the care and service Mom was receiving. Mom explained that her main concern was the frustration of meal requests not being fulfilled, and she was assured this would be taken care of. Mom was relieved. Unfortunately, this was not the case, and meals continued to be a problem. She experienced a number of other inefficiencies during her five-day stay, which she found irritating. Being a healthcare management and marketing consultant, I drew a distinguishing line between management's desire to implement a superior customer service program and its inability to implement it effectively throughout the organization. It was obvious that not everyone in this hospital was on board with the *Pampered Guest* campaign.

Analysis

1. The organization launched its new customer service program prematurely.
2. The organization failed to get program buy-in from all stakeholders.
3. There was not enough attention given to the implementation.
4. Channels of communication were weak.
5. Unfulfilled campaign promises exacerbated patient frustration and negatively influenced patient satisfaction.

Having a vision for and establishing a customer service initiative is likely to result in embarrassment and disappointing results if the culture of the organization has a history it must overcome in order to change attitudes and behavior it has not dealt with first. You must develop a shared customer service culture of respect as a first step to developing effective processes to change the organization's culture and test it long before you launch an ambitious promise to provide superior customer service.

This hospital needed to make sure everyone shared a service culture—and it started at the top! If the leaders of the organization do not honor and respect the people that report directly to them, they cannot expect the employees that serve the patients to be patient-centered. The nurse who bristled at my mother and me most likely did not feel valued by her supervisor, or she and her peers did not feel they would be held accountable if they neglected to respond to a patient's needs. The social worker that felt burdened and didn't even have her own computer could not be expected to be confident that she could meet the needs of the patients that were assigned to her, no matter how much she wanted to. Rolling out a customer service program when these problems exist is bound to result in failure.

Outcome

Because I was not working with this hospital, I wasn't privy to the strategies and objectives of the Pampered Guest program or the politics involved. I was not in a position to make professional recommendations or help it take corrective actions to overcome the dilemma that was created by the premature rollout of the Pampered Guest program. However, being naturally curious because of my profession, I walked through the hospital on one of my visits to Mom a year later. There were no signs of the Pampered Guest program. I made a telephone inquiry and was told the program was on hold and being revamped. I don't wonder why. It is unfortunate a good idea wasn't successfully executed, and it cost the hospital substantial resources. In the end, the hospital's shortcomings were magnified through a program that was likely meant to increase its patient satisfaction scores.

CASE STUDY

Good Wasn't Good Enough

Malcolm Ellison, MD, strategically positioned his pediatric practice in a suburban neighborhood in a town that had plenty of pediatricians on the other side of town but none in the secluded neighborhood full of young families that would be thrilled to have their child's doctor along the same route they took to the grocery store and schools. He placed an ad in the local paper, opened his doors, and waited for the flood of patients; instead he got a trickle. After a couple of months of miniscule growth, he called us in specifically for marketing to build his patient base. He didn't have the budget for a strategic marketing plan, so we prepared a list of marketing actions that we knew would get his practice rolling.

We developed the practice image to fit Dr. Ellison's personality and style, and used thoughtful and provoking copy to tell potential patients why they should confidently choose him. We reached out to the community in ways that fit the mission and image of the practice and made Dr. Ellison visible on many fronts including the Internet.

Dr. Ellison was fortunate to have started out with a strong idea of customer service in regard to how staff should speak to patients and the technology patients' expected, including electronic health records, a patient portal, and automated reminder calls. He also had a relaxed yet respectful bedside manner that patients trusted. Combined with a commitment to commonsense marketing, these elements were a recipe for success. Soon the patient numbers grew, and Dr. Ellison breathed a sigh of relief as he watched the practice grow . . . and grow. He began to add staff members who offered the same great customer service as his original team, and before long he was interviewing a second provider.

Everything seemed to be going as planned until the numbers flat-lined. Dr. Ellison knew that the demographics of the community should keep his services in high demand, yet he couldn't quite get the patient load up to potential for both him and the new provider, Carrie Devereaux, NP. Patients seemed to have a good rapport with both of them and the staff; the office was very conveniently located; and, though minimally, he was still promoting the practice and keeping his name in front of potential and existing patients. Referrals from existing patients weren't as strong as he'd hoped, and he was perplexed by the lack of demand in a community that seemed to really need the practice's services.

It was then that we took a deeper look at the practice operating policies that might impact patient service and possible nuances of the patient experience from the perspective of the patients' life-style needs. Through this assessment and the power of third-party surveying and interviewing patients, we were able to pinpoint some areas that the physician and staff had never considered to be of any "serious concern."

Dr. Ellison considered his practice to be *one of the best* as far as customer service and patient-centeredness went. He had heard horror stories of practices that were unorganized, unfriendly, and out of touch with new technologies. He knew his practice was a cut above *those kinds* of practices, and any complaints or suggestions he got were weighed against the majority of complimentary comments from happy patients and then dismissed.

What Dr. Ellison didn't realize is that unhappy patients seldom say anything to their doctor; and if they do speak up, they are more likely to tell the staff. And it is even more uncommon for employees to let the physician know about the complaint. When patients like their healthcare provider, they are hesitant to be honest about the disappointing aspects of their experience with the practice—not wanting to be seen as a complainer or ungrateful.

We found three ways the practice was falling short in meeting the needs of their patients—or their parents, in this case.

When patients called in at noon, or 12:30, or 1:00, they had to leave a message on voicemail because the office was closed from 12:00 PM to 1:30 PM. Not trusting that their message was heard and being responded to, and often distressed about an ailing child, parents would call back again after the lunch hour and be greeted by an overwhelmed staff that couldn't confirm whether their previous message had been addressed or not. This lack of ability to communicate with the practice at midday caused distress for working parents whose lunch hour was the ideal time to make phone calls regarding their child's healthcare, as well as for those seeking immediate care for a child who was sent home early from school.

Although we have strong convictions about the importance of keeping phone lines open during business hours, we wanted to explore how other practices in the community were managing phones during lunch. In other words, was Dr. Ellison's policy consistent with that of his competition? We discovered that some practices offered phone coverage during the midday lunch hour, and some did not. This placed Dr. Ellison's practice on the *less patient-friendly* side of the equation. Additional research revealed that parents of pediatric patients would highly value the ability to be seen on a Saturday, whether for a sudden illness or a regular vaccination that could be taken care of without taking time off from work.

We also found that patients felt *nickeled and dimed* when they needed copies of a vaccination card or health record, or if they missed an appointment. The charges they incurred felt punitive and were breaking down the trust and loyalty that Dr. Ellison and his staff were working so hard to build with their warm in-person communication with patients in the office. Most of these parents had no desire to miss an appointment for their child; but in the busy world of parenting multiple children and holding down jobs and maintaining extracurricular schedules, sometimes a well visit would be forgotten. Being charged a fee on top of their own disappointment for missing the visit or every time they needed a doctor's signature on a school form wasn't encouraging them to send their friends to the practice.

The last issue we uncovered was very practical and would seem obvious except to those who don't walk through the practice as the patient on a day-in and day-out basis. The reception room was small, uncomfortable, and unaccommodating to the needs of the parents toting strollers, toddlers, and otherwise wily kiddos. The space was simply too small and made bringing the stroller along very awkward, so parents learned to leave it in the car—except that many of Dr. Ellison's patients were able to walk to his office from home, a great advantage but a huge inconvenience when it came to the stroller. The chairs were hard and uncomfortable with no cushions, and the lovely water feature Dr. Ellison had installed before opening his practice was a huge temptation for the little ones, causing parents to have to work diligently during the entire wait to keep their kids from making a complete mess.

Analysis

1. By shutting down phones during the lunch hour, the practice was inaccessible to patients during nearly 20% of normal business hours.

2. No objective patient satisfaction surveys had been conducted.
3. The practice was unaware of how much patients would appreciate Saturday hours.
4. The reception room had a décor that did not provide comfort for patients and was ill equipped for young children.
5. The reception area did not accommodate strollers, thus presenting a problem for parents who traveled on foot from nearby neighborhoods.
6. The policy of charging for missed appointments and copies of vaccination records was felt by patients to be punitive. The cost to the practice to bill and collect payment far exceeded these fees.

Our observations and analysis revealed some problems that could be easily fixed, but Dr. Ellison was surprised that these seemingly small issues could weigh so heavily on the growth of his practice. It is often a subconscious feeling or thought process on the part of your patients, but these practical issues make a strong impact on whether or not your practice gives your patients something special—enough to establish loyalty and get their tongues wagging to their friends so that you reap excited referrals! Dr. Ellison had heard all of these issues brought up at some time in the past, but because patients weren't angry and the issues weren't mentioned repeatedly, he didn't realize how much of an impact they had on patients. Research indicates[1] that for every one customer who complains there are 25 others that remain silent; they often simply take their business elsewhere. For this reason, negative feedback can be your best friend—it gives you an opportunity to sharpen your practice and rise above the competition.

Recommendations

1. Keep phones open during all business hours by staggering staff lunches.
2. Extend office hours to include a limited Saturday morning clinic with alternate providers and creative support staff scheduling.
3. Eliminate nominal charges for missed appointments and providing vaccination records.

4. Provide comfortable seating and a child-friendly environment in the reception room.
5. Provide an area for stroller parking.
6. Improve patient feedback by installing a suggestion box and conducting an annual patient survey.

Outcome

We approached the implementation by addressing the easiest fixes first. We began by providing a suggestion box in the reception area where patients could anonymously give sincere feedback. Additionally, an annual e-mailed patient survey was conducted to provide feedback on specific quality and satisfaction measurements.

The practice eliminated the fees that patients found to be annoying. We took a proactive approach to reduce missed appointments by creating scripts for staff that emphasize to patients the importance of keeping their appointments. We also determined that a part-time employee paid minimum wage could easily manage the demand for copies of vaccination records, thereby reducing response time and the time that staff members were distracted with these requests. This increased staff efficiency and reduced costs while improving patient satisfaction. Additionally, we began to research automated online immunization registries that would eliminate this labor-intensive process that did not generate revenue.

Maintaining lunch hour phone coverage by staggering staff lunch breaks improved patient service and eliminated the afternoon crunch previously caused by peak demands on phones. Repeat calls and post-lunch stress were reduced, and efficiency and telephone access were markedly improved.

An open area was identified in the building's pharmacy that was ideal for stroller parking. This brought welcome foot traffic to the pharmacy increasing its sales and provided a much-appreciated service to Dr. Ellison's patients.

Each provider scheduled one Saturday morning clinic each month. The practice found this to be extremely popular with patients and eventually one provider took over this position in exchange for a Friday off each month.

Comfortable seating was purchased for the reception room, which now included fun activities and a safe décor for children. The fountain was moved to the employee lounge.

After six months, patient satisfaction ratings soared, and referrals increased. With improved efficiency and glowing remarks from patients, staff and providers felt far more fulfilled. They were pleased with all the improvements that were made and believed they were better prepared for future growth. The most important change we initiated was improving the practice culture to match the customer service-oriented mission of this pediatric practice. Now the practice is listening to patients and truly meeting their needs in ways that exceed patient expectations—thus setting it apart from the competition and deepening patient loyalty.

CASE STUDY
Not So Warm and Fuzzy

Marcia Taylor, MD, contacted us when she felt overwhelmed with her solo OB/GYN practice operations. She had been in private practice for the past four years and experienced rapid growth, but things weren't going the way she expected. She knew her purpose and delighted in building the practice of her dreams. Now each day started off smoothly, but it ended with confusion, stress, and exhaustion. Patient flow had become a major problem, even though she had five exam rooms. She just couldn't keep up with the patient load and would fall behind by end of each morning and afternoon session. Patient service was being sacrificed. Our goal was to determine the root cause of the problem and help the practice create a smooth-running day that was consistent with living its mission.

Dr. Taylor's mission would make any aspiring mother swoon; "*To touch lives with compassionate, personal care; one woman, one mother, one baby at a time.*" She was so passionate about her mission that her staff was required to gather every morning, before any patients arrived, to review the mission and declare a daily mantra that would inspire them in achieving it. They held hands and shared warm thoughts, a moment of peace before the demands of serving a bustling practice full of expectant mothers. Dr. Taylor and her nurse practitioner, Deborah Bechtel, NP, were well known and loved in their community—patients loved how they were looked in the eye and listened to during visits. When a patient longing to become pregnant finally received the good news, the staff quickly gathered around her in congratulations to give a gift and a group hurrah.

There is no doubt Dr. Taylor was exemplary in her desire and commitment to connect and provide emotionally for her patients. On a table in the hallway were framed photos of their patients' babies who had survived against uncommonly great odds. There were inspirational plaques throughout the facility seemingly communicating, "We believe in miracles, we won't give up on you." Dr. Taylor felt a deep satisfaction with her connection to her patients.

In spite of her rewarding patient relationships and having a staff she felt confident in, Dr. Taylor sensed an underlying dysfunction within the practice that she couldn't quite put her finger on. By 2:00 PM each day, chaos would begin to rule. The upbeat bustle of the morning would turn into a more frantic flurry. Dr. Taylor worked very hard to serve both her obstetric and gynecology patients and create the most positive work environment possible, and she had the support of her nurse practitioner to help with prenatal visits and instructions, yet she knew something just wasn't right.

We were brought in to assess practice efficiency. Before arriving onsite, considerable data were requested and reviewed to help us become familiar with the practice's current position. We began the onsite assessment with a tour of the facility, followed by observation and interviews with the employees. It was important to understand their perspective on the practice and its service, and what issues they believed were relevant to our engagement. It was clear that the employees admired Dr. Taylor, what she stood for, and how she was revered by her loyal patients. Unfortunately, this didn't translate into the relationship between the employees and the physician.

We interviewed each employee and discovered two of them were new, having come on board within the past few weeks. They had very little training in a very busy office and didn't understand their role or what was expected of them. They felt unimportant and inadequate. Suzanne was the checkout receptionist. However, she was also required to back up the check-in receptionist. When checking-in patients, she knew what information to collect but didn't know how to update demographics on the computer. Everyone was so busy, they didn't have time to show her. She was worried she would make a mistake, and the work kept piling up. Suzanne was required to handle all inbound calls at the checkout station. When patients called in to schedule an appointment, the next available opening was three weeks away. When patients needed to be seen sooner, she didn't know what to do. In order to pacify the caller, she took down the person's phone number and said someone would get back to her. She knew this was compromising patient service, and it made her very uncomfortable, but didn't know what else to do.

The obstetric patients being seen weekly would request their next appointment when checking out; and, again, there were no open appointments at the time they needed to be seen. Patients would get angry, and Suzanne would buzz the office manager who then took over and scheduled the patient. Unfortunately, this meant double booking, which presented another issue with wait times when patients arrived in the office the next week.

During our interview with Suzanne, she revealed that she desperately needed this job, but knew she couldn't perform well under the circumstances and without proper training. She was terrified a patient would ask her a question she didn't have the answer to and was feeling incompetent. She was even more terrified she would be fired because of this.

Dianna, the other new employee, was an experienced biller who had inherited a major problem. The previous biller left a month before

Dianna was hired, and the work had been neglected. The phone was constantly ringing with patients that received statements with errors on them, and the statements didn't specify whether the patients' insurance had been billed. Dianna was unflappable and just went about correcting problems and giving every person she talked to good service. She just took control. Unfortunately, this meant she was making policy and procedure decisions on the fly without approval. It made sense to her because the manager didn't know anything about billing. Dianna wasn't given any guidelines or written procedures when she was hired. She thought she was doing a great job because she was seeing the results of her hard work by rapidly improving cash flow and reducing accounts receivable.

Dianna was a dedicated employee, but she also had little communication with other staff members. During our interview, she made a point of telling us there was no interaction between her and Dr. Taylor, but felt it didn't impede her work. It was obvious that she was a good employee—a self-starter with a strong work ethic—but she needed guidance to avoid making decisions that required approval from the physician, such as changing CPT codes on several services because the codes she used would improve reimbursement.

Other staff members loved being a part of the practice as well. Most of them had joined the practice in the beginning, back when Dr. Taylor had time to spend with employees. It was then that Dr. Taylor decided that, though atypical, she'd prefer to manage her staff because she felt the relationships she built with staff were crucial to living out her mission. She wanted to stay connected and understand what each person was contributing to the practice. For this reason, her office manager was less involved in staff supervision and performance issues, focusing more on administrative responsibilities.

Dr. Taylor's approach made long-time staff members feel valued and loyal to the practice. They seemed to accept that things changed with growth and knew she didn't have an idle moment, but they longed for the *good old days* when there was much more interaction.

Dr. Taylor was busy moving from patient to patient and from the office to the hospital. She no longer had time to talk with staff beyond the passing pleasantries of being courteous. She was preoccupied with staying on time and moving through a jam-packed day. She was so focused that she didn't have time to engage the employees. This type of situation can be confusing and intimidating to new employees. It was a dichotomy: patients raving about the doctor while new employees were feeling ignored, insignificant, and abandoned.

The patient flow did indeed compromise patient service and cause stress throughout the office. Filling five exam rooms at one time in order to empty the reception area gave staff a feeling of being *caught-up*, but Dr. Taylor knew better. The physician might be treating a patient in one room and a nurse might be taking care of another, but that still left three patients stuck waiting in small exam rooms without the comfort of back-supporting chairs and distractions to help the time pass, having already changed into a gown and growing ever-more aware that the physician was making them wait. Anticipating an expected 15 minutes for each visit meant it would be at least 45 minutes before the doctor would be greeting the patient now being roomed by the nurse. This was not the experience she wanted for her patients, especially for the obstetric patients who could be very uncomfortable.

Staff was double-booking patients because of the excessive demand, and this just exacerbated a problem that was already unmanageable. This was a recipe for disaster and was contrary to Dr. Taylor's beliefs and her mission of providing compassionate and personal care. No wonder she didn't have time to connect with staff. Even her interaction with clinical staff was minimal. She was like a whirlwind when she was in the office.

Analysis

Dr. Taylor had a heart of gold and enjoyed her patients immensely. She also believed she had a fantastic staff. The problem was she was so busy and overwhelmed that patients were beginning to feel shortchanged. The new staff members were falling through the cracks as well. They considered it a privilege to work for Dr. Taylor, considering her incredible reputation among patients and medical staff in the community, but they found themselves feeling disconnected and disappointed. They got the impression that there had been a more joyful time in the practice, and those long-term employees experienced and remembered it and knew Dr. Taylor for who she was then, but new employees didn't share those experiences or know her that way.

The scheduling and workflow appeared to be the cause for these hectic and out-of-control days, but the real root of the problem was excessive demand with too little access. Dr. Taylor didn't want to turn away any new patient from the bustling practice she'd grown, yet it was impossible to meet the demand without paying a price. Unfortunately that price was compromising the ability to live the mission she felt so passionate about and sapping the joy out of the workplace. It was changing the culture of the practice, and *everyone* was feeling it.

It was time to regroup and look at the potential solutions to solve this dilemma. She needed to focus on ways to meet the patients' demand and keep satisfaction high. She also needed to find time to communicate better with her staff. We could help her address and solve the scheduling issues to control workflow better with strategic scheduling, but to fully meet demand, we provided Dr. Taylor with two options to consider:
1. Limit acceptance of new patients; or
2. Bring in another provider.

Recommendations

1. Determine whether to limit acceptance of new patients and keep it small, or add another physician to meet the existing and growing demand.
2. Once the above decision is made, begin the processes necessary to accomplish it.
3. Examine and clarify practice goals for the next 12 to 24 months.
4. Conduct a staff meeting and discuss:
   a. The priorities of the mission;

  b. Practice goals and objectives (based on #1 above); and

  c. A plan to renew the culture of connectedness and joy the practice once experienced.

5. Develop a reasonable template for the appointment schedule to accommodate existing patient load.

   a. Eliminate double-booking;

   b. Hold enough weekly appointments to accommodate obstetric patients during the last six weeks of their prenatal care; and

   c. Develop a group (shared) appointment for obstetric patients in the month following their initial workup. Most patients love this group setting and sharing the excitement about having a baby. For the practice, it creates more individual time on the schedule.

6. Schedule the physician to have a 25-minute mini-conference with the manager and each new employee weekly during the employee's first month on the job to provide support, encouragement, and further orientation; build the relationship; and monitor the employee's progress.

Outcome

Dr. Taylor decided to add another provider to help meet the existing scheduling demands. Within six weeks, she was able to find a nurse practitioner, Shari Wong, with experience in women's health who was excited to join a physician with such an incredible respect and passion for her patients. They clicked immediately.

After adding the nurse practitioner, the double-bookings came to a halt, and a new scheduling template was created. It provided the scheduler with the ability to reserve adequate appointments for those weekly obstetric patients during the last six weeks of their pregnancy. And with Shari's help, they were easily prepared to accommodate annual physicals that were previously being delayed. They even began to offer evening appointments once a week to accommodate patients who found it difficult to keep appointments during regular business hours.

The practice also began the recruitment process to add another OB-GYN physician—a process that can easily take up to a year. Over a period of three months, we reviewed more than 40 *curricula vitae* and selected 20 to conduct telephone interviews with. This resulted in selecting nine physicians for Dr. Taylor and us to interview. Some of them were Skype interviews because they were living in other parts of the country. After properly vetting these applicants, a selection was made, and we offered the position to a physician who was completing her fellowship. We entered contract negotiations and scheduled a start date three months later.

Before long, this practice was back on track. The new providers and added support staff embraced the mission, and the patient experience was greatly improved. The practice was growing in leaps and bounds, the camaraderie was contagious, the energy was palpable, and the employees were living the mission.

COMMON THREAD

The common thread in these case studies is cultural differences or shifts that impede patient service. Your organization's internal culture influences everything from the first impression to lasting impressions that dramatically affect your patients' experience. Staff members often become preoccupied with the technical components of their job and the task of staying on schedule. When this happens, it's easy to fall short in providing the personal connection that yields stellar reviews and patient loyalty. However, when staff members understand how important their roles are in making that connection, and the culture of the practice reinforces this goal, you *can* succeed!

GETTING THERE

The administrative leaders of your organization must be committed to the mission of providing an excellent patient experience. The more passionate leaders are and the more they communicate that conviction to the staff, the more excited and authentic the staff buy-in will be. Your staff members must understand how important their role is in giving quality service as you develop methods to hold them accountable and reward success.

Here is a list of actionable items you can apply immediately to help turn your healthcare organization's culture around, or simply take it up a notch:

1. Invest time in developing a plan to align your staff's commitment with the mission—to share your vision and goal.

2. Treat staff members properly—they are your first customer. If they are not treated with respect and courtesy, you cannot expect them to give patients a caring experience based on respect, honor, and commitment.

3. Create patient service performance standards that are measurable for each position, particularly those that come in contact with and serve the patients. Remember, however, that even your maintenance people should be trained to smile and say hello to anyone passing by, and to offer assistance if someone looks as if he or she is in need of help or is lost. This speaks volumes about an organization's customer service commitment.

4. Use the service standards for each position as a component of the employee's annual performance review and compensation gains. For example, if one standard is that the receptionist and nurse must introduce themselves to each new patient, an observation or survey process must take place to ensure this is happening consistently.

5. Dedicate resources to develop customer service programs for new staff members that include a discussion about their individual performance standards and how these are a key part of the performance review process.

6. Measure patient satisfaction, and pay attention to how results change over time—but be sure you are willing to take corrective action when the marks are not to your satisfaction.

7. Conduct annual staff refresher courses on customer service, and review how well your organization is performing and meeting its patient service goals.
8. When developing initiatives, involve staff by asking for suggestions and giving them serious consideration.
9. Share your success, and honor everyone's contribution. Celebrations energize and reaffirm your shared patient-centered culture.

These steps will lead to a better understanding of everyone's contribution, and provide a culture of shared values, aligning your entire organization for success!

THE PAYOFF

When healthcare leaders are in sync with their mission and display the organization's core values, the impact is so powerful that it's almost impossible not to succeed. Your organization's internal culture influences first and lasting impressions that dramatically affect your patients' experience while providing the foundation for a cohesive staff environment that is deeply satisfying.

Reference

1. Wysocki A, Kepner K, Galsser M. Customer Complains and Types of Customers. Document HR005. Institute of Food and Agricultural Sciences, University of Florida, Reviewed 2012; http://edis.ifas.ufl.edu/hr005.

CHAPTER 6

Cultural Differences: When Hospitals Own Practices

By Coauthor Judy Capko

I was called into a well-known, respected hospital system to conduct assessments of several practices it had acquired within the prior year. None of these practices had made the adjustment to hospital ownership that was expected. Performance and patient service suffered. Satisfaction was at an all-time low for physicians, staff, and patients. Confusion about the relationship between the hospital and the practices resulted in deteriorating service and attitudes. The case studies presented in this chapter offer a perfect example of how the best intentions don't always bring the best results and how cultural differences can be at the root of a healthcare organization's most daunting problems.

Tri-City Hospital was concerned about the performance of three medical practices it recently acquired. My consulting assignment was to provide an objective analysis of these practices, clarify the primary issues of concern, and provide recommendations that would guide the hospital to:

1. Overcome obstacles causing poor performance, deteriorating morale, and poor patient satisfaction; and

2. Resolve conflicts between the hospital and these medical practices.

CASE STUDY

Misery Is Contagious: Community Family Clinic

Community Family Clinic consisted of three internists, five family physicians, and two nurse practitioners. They were well-suited to practice together, sharing common values; they worked with a motivated staff; and the finances were solid. But over the past few years, they started feeling the demands of more regulatory requirements, flat reimbursement, and expectations that the impact of healthcare reform posed a threat to the practice's finances and stability. The physicians began to question their future security. The privilege of owning the practice was beginning to feel like a burden. They didn't believe they had the business expertise to deal with the unknown changes required with healthcare reform or the potential consequences it would bring to their practice. They began to question their future security.

The timing seemed ideal when the hospital approached the physicians about this primary care clinic joining the hospital and the physicians becoming hospital employees. Surely the hospital had far greater resources and business acumen to help them ride the waves of reform without economic disaster! The clinic already resided on the hospital's campus, making the merger even more appealing. After a few discussions and deliberate planning and with the aid of lawyers and accountants, they joined forces. It wasn't long before the practice was acquired and functioning under the Tri-City Hospital banner. The physicians breathed a sigh of relief, but not everyone was happy.

I met with Anthony Costello, the practice administrator, to begin the onsite engagement with a briefing of Community Family Clinic's history and an overview of its current position. Anthony had been with the practice for seven years and was instrumental in the practice's continual growth and financial stability during his tenure. When the hospital began courting the practice, he wasn't terribly concerned, as the physicians kept him informed throughout the process. It seemed the hospital's plans were to have the practice continue under its current operations management and work toward a seamless transition. The hospital was straightforward with its plan for Community Family Clinic to convert to the hospital's practice management billing system and also stated that the staff would be employed by the hospital, providing the employees with an appealing benefits package. The physicians and Anthony were assured that staff positions would remain unchanged even though the staff members would be working for the hospital.

Six weeks before the deal closing, Anthony asked to meet with the hospital's vice president of human resources to develop a staff plan and to clarify his own future responsibilities. He became concerned when excuses were made and no meeting was set. He not only wanted to understand what was expected of him, but he also wanted his staff members to have a clear picture of what they could expect and what support they would receive from the hospital. That never happened. It seems the integration plan did not give enough attention to communicating with staff members, making them feel important, and clarifying what would change once the hospital took ownership of the practice.

Anthony knew working with the hospital would entail a more structured business model, but he was not prepared for the cultural shift required and the impact it would have on the entire practice. Staff members were given new boilerplate job descriptions that were vague and meaningless. The end result was the employees felt disconnected from their new employer. As frustration mounted, an attitude of *"us versus them"* became prevalent within the clinic. The additional red tape required to comply with hospital standards just added to the challenges and frustration of the workplace. Anthony understood he would need to provide productivity and management reports, but believed the reports fell into a big black hole since there was no discussion about how these reports were used and no feedback on the practice's performance. For his own purposes, he kept tracking performance using the internal benchmarks he was accustomed to using before the practice joined the hospital, but this was not information the hospital showed any interest in.

The employees unanimously complained that the hospital didn't care about them or understand how hard they worked. The hospital kept asking more of them without providing additional resources. For example, because it was a provider-based practice working for the hospital, there were far more regulatory issues that needed to be followed and forms the patients were required to complete. The staff members were not told why they needed to get these forms completed, so when the patients complained, the staff would just blame the hospital. The billers now worked at the hospital and weren't available at the practice to answer questions from patients or staff. Staff members didn't know how much money to collect from patients and weren't prepared to answer billing questions. Patients were complaining and didn't know where to turn.

Staff members were also not happy with the practice management system they felt they were forced to use and were poorly trained to do so. The scheduling module was labor-intensive, and the data entry process was not user-friendly. The system frequently locked up, and cries for help to the hospital's IT department seemed to fall on deaf ears. To top it off, Anthony was spending more time in meetings at the hospital now, making him less available to his own staff. He had understood the hospital would require more of him, but wasn't prepared for the amount of time it would require him to be offsite and the seemingly endless rounds of meetings he would need to attend. The employees felt ignored, and Anthony felt guilty.

CASE STUDY

Unrealistic Expectations: Orthopaedic Associates

The hospital approached Orthopaedic Associates, a three-physician orthopaedic practice, a year ago with what seemed like an offer the physicians couldn't refuse. The practice had outgrown its office space, which was dreadfully outdated, and the physicians were tired of schlepping to and from the hospital, seven miles from their office. The hospital proposal was very appealing, with an offer to provide Orthopaedic Associates with a brand-new office suite on the hospital campus. It would be attached to an ambulatory surgery center (ASC) and an imaging center.

The physicians began to imagine how convenient this would be: how it would save them the cost of relocating to a bigger facility by themselves, offer seamless convenience for their patients, and give the practice an edge over the competition. They dreamed about all their problems going away with a guaranteed income and the hospital's business-savvy administrators at the helm.

Within a few months the deal was complete, and their new facility was under construction. They moved into the new office three months before my visit, but things weren't going as they anticipated.

My first meeting was with the practice manager, Rebecca Sage. The doctors and staff used her as a sounding board to vent all their complaints. The new space was nice, but the physicians who were accustomed to large consultation rooms were now in smaller offices with additional workspace adjoining the nurses' station. They complained about the lack of privacy and said they were constantly interrupted and unable to get their work done. Nurses complained that the doctors were becoming antagonistic, and there was some in-fighting. Rebecca felt hamstrung when it came to getting approval from the hospital to make changes. "It takes an act of Congress to get decisions made," she said, lamenting the good old days when if a doctor wanted a new piece of equipment it would be discussed at the practice's monthly meeting and ordered within a short period of time.

In addition, there was a change in attitude displayed by one of the physicians since the move. Dr. Jenkins was clearly frustrated with the hospital's constant interference with how the practice was managed and its seeming criticism of everyone's performance, and the highly structured business model the physicians now worked under. As her frustration continued to mount, she began to ignore it all, doing her own thing. She was viewed as a maverick by much of the practice team. She was out of sync with everyone in the practice and was starting to bristle with the patients. She was clearly unhappy, but wasn't talking about it. She just took more time off and saw fewer patients when she was in the office. Dr. Jenkins' productivity plummeted. She was consistently delayed in returning from the hospital, causing her to run late, and patients were complaining. The scheduler was frustrated because Dr. Jenkins wanted a lighter schedule when demand was already greater than capacity.

It was an impossible situation. Dr. Jenkins seemed generally disconnected from the practice. Her patients were bolting. Some were demanding to switch to one of the other physicians, whose schedules were already at capacity, and others were leaving the practice altogether. These three physicians who had gotten along well for years were now at odds with each other. The hospital was holding the practice responsible for Dr. Jenkins' behavior, and her two partners were justifiably upset.

So was Rebecca. She was a conscientious self-starter with a record for being a top performer, but was beginning to feel a sense of helplessness, believing she had more responsibilities than she could possibly handle and a dismal support system. Rebecca was now required to manage both the orthopaedic practice and the hospital's newly acquired gastroenterology practice, Anderson Digestive Medicine. She was struggling for acceptance from the new practice's existing staff. Her workload was far more demanding with running two practices and the new responsibilities the hospital placed on her. Even though she was no longer responsible for billing, she was the one that had to handle billing questions that came up when patients were in the office for an appointment. Many of these patients were confused, not fully understanding the connection with the hospital and getting billing statements that were totally unfamiliar to them. Rebecca felt like she was drowning and, like Anthony, was being called into administrative meetings at the hospital that further decreased her ability to give either practice the management attention it deserved.

CASE STUDY

A Sense of Abandonment: Anderson Digestive Medicine

Donald Anderson, MD, ran a busy solo gastroenterology practice with a full-time nurse practitioner. He also owned the adjoining ASC, where he spent most mornings doing procedures. He was working at capacity and in the process of recruiting another gastroenterologist when the hospital approached him about acquiring his practice. It offered to take over the recruitment of a new physician and the associated costs. It also wanted to purchase the ASC and release him from the responsibility of managing both the ASC and his practice.

Dr. Anderson was tired of the business side of medicine, and he welcomed the opportunity to join the hospital and follow suit with some of the other physicians in the community. His office manager was planning to retire, and he was assured the hospital's management team would be able to provide the practice with a higher level of business management expertise, leaving him free to focus entirely on the clinical side of the practice. What he didn't realize was that the small practice culture would disappear once the hospital was running the show. The camaraderie of the small practice environment and the freedom in how he managed staff decisions changed in ways he had not anticipated.

Employees felt like "Big Brother" was watching them. They didn't like that the hospital's human resources department gave them new job descriptions and would be involved in when and how they would receive performance reviews. The employees resented what they perceived to be a lot of unnecessary paperwork and red tape. Dr. Anderson hadn't realized the ASC would be independent of the practice and be staffed by hospital personnel. This left Dr. Anderson with a smaller staff that felt totally disconnected from its previous team members at the ASC. Dr. Anderson was also less involved in how patient care was managed at the ASC. The staff members missed the good old days and complained about how the hospital burdened them with more work, hadn't replaced their full-time manager, and seemed to show little interest in the workings of their practice operations.

Rebecca Sage, managing this practice as well as Orthopaedic Associates, spent very little time in the office. The hospital's administrator was always asking for a variety of management reports, but didn't give her a clue as to why. Rebecca had no idea how the practice was measuring up and didn't really know what the hospital expected when it came to the practice's performance.

CONSULTANT'S OVERVIEW

The overarching problem between the hospital and these three practices was without question a clash of cultures and too little attention to building trust and developing shared goals and a plan to achieve them. Unrealistic expectations and weak channels of communication further compromised the relationship between the hospital and the practices (Figure 1).

Without question, there were unrealistic expectations on both sides of this equation. The hospital clearly did not have an understanding of how small medical practices function, and the practices had unrealistic expectations of the support they would receive from the hospital. These practices did not have

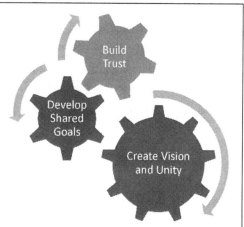

FIGURE 1. Overcoming the cultural clash between the hospital and the practice.

a clear vision of how the practice operations would change under hospital ownership and gave little thought to what the hospital's goals were in acquiring them. The three practices did not understand the restrictions and regulatory issues the hospital would require them to abide by. They also didn't understand the reason for all of the red tape and time required to make changes and obtain approval for requests. All these factors created barriers to building trust and creating a unified front.

Analysis

The hospital did an admirable job with vetting the practices financially and managing the legal and financial requirements in acquiring these practices and developing a governance plan. This was no small accomplishment and required considerable resources, both administrative and financial, to complete successfully. Unfortunately, too little attention was given to gaining an understanding of the culture and mindset of small practices that were accustomed to making quick business and financial decisions, even though those decisions were sometimes reactive. In the hospital, such decisions often required considerable investigation and administrative discussion, and an organizational hierarchical process.

These three medical practices were previously managed in a more casual manner than that of the hospital. There was limited organizational structure, policies and procedures were not well-defined, and in fact only one of the practices had formal job descriptions for the staff. The physicians and staff did not realize how difficult it would be to adjust to a more structured business model.

These issues were immobilizing the hospital's ability to build trust and create unity between it and the practices it now owned. It needed the physician leaders and practice managers to be part of the solution. Below are the major issues that contributed to the friction and dissatisfaction that were festering within these provider-based practices and the performance issues that concerned the hospital's administrative team:

1. No shared vision;
2. Failure to create unity between hospital administration and the medical practices;
3. Inadequate staff integration plan;
4. Lack of physician performance benchmarks and clear productivity expectations;
5. Failure to develop effective channels of communication;
6. Limited support from the hospital's human resources department;
7. Disconnect between the hospital's human resources department and the practices;
8. Poor morale; and
9. Dissatisfied patients.

Recommendations

Our goal was to focus on improving communication, creating unity through a strategic process that would identify shared goals and negotiate how these goals would be achieved and what would be required of each key stakeholder to accomplish them:

1. Schedule a strategic retreat, planned and facilitated by the consulting team.
2. Develop a strategic plan to:
   a. Determine the shared vision;
   b. Establish specific goals; and
   c. Assign appropriate responsibilities.
3. Create and maintain operational unity by:
   a. Conducting a meeting with the hospital team, physicians, and each practice administrator to discuss the findings of

my assessment and recommended approach to resolving existing problems and providing a more promising future;

b. Establishing a work session with the practice administrators, hospital physician liaison, and the vice president of human resources to develop a staff integration plan for each practice, clarifying what support would be provided to the staff by the hospital; and

c. Developing cross-functional teams to guide and participate in the following actions:

    i. Distribute a job description questionnaire for each staff member to complete in order to prepare more accurate job descriptions;

    ii. Prepare a training guide for each position based on the new job descriptions;

    iii. Develop key performance indicators for each position that will be used as a performance metric during the employee's performance reviews;

    iv. Schedule monthly staff meetings for each practice; and

    v. Schedule quarterly combined staff meetings with all managers and appropriate hospital administrative participants.

Outcome

After reviewing my report and determining the most practical approach to achieve the organizational goals, there were a number of executive staff meetings. A timeline was developed to approach implementing the recommendations. The ultimate goal was to develop a trusting relationship between the executive team of the hospital and the medical practices it acquired. This required developing shared goals and creating a work plan based on mutual input that would build unity and develop solid work teams with a shared purpose.

LESSONS LEARNED

Unrealistic expectations and a failure to understand the importance of cultural differences between hospitals and medical practices often result in division and failure to unite. In this situation, the problem was addressed early on, and changes were made before the hospital reached out to other physicians to become part of its organization.

Understanding cultural differences when bringing different groups and entities into a collaborative partnership is critical. Culture is the heart of each organization—its beliefs and what it stands for. Integrating cultural beliefs into a future partnership can only happen if those beliefs and ethics are aligned with those of the potential partners. It is important to start the partnership process by having honest discussions and gaining an understanding of what each stake-holder thinks it will gain from the partnership and understanding each other's intentions. What are their goals; what do they hope to achieve; and, just as importantly, what will each of them give that will make the partnership stronger, and what will the merged group gain? It is through this process that each person can make the best decision; and when a person chooses to come on board, he or she will contribute to building trust and unity.

Finally, physicians who are accustomed to being the owner and making their own practice decisions are sometimes challenged with the new business arrangement. They can sometimes become disconnected from the strategic planning and financial requirements essential to sustaining the hospital-owned, provider-based practice. The relationship between a hospital and the medical practices it acquires calls for a clear delineation of responsibilities and expectations, as well as defined performance goals.

THE PAYOFF

The relationship between a hospital and the medical practices it acquires calls for a clear delineation of responsibilities, expectations, and performance goals in order to address cultural differences that may exist. By setting these in place ahead of time, the organization can head off frustration, disillusionment, and disengagement while building trust, respect, shared values, and common goals for success.

CHAPTER 7

Conflicts on the Patient-Centered Journey

Healthcare professionals, buried in a myriad of work problems and facing the demands of healthcare reform, have reason to be concerned. How can they keep up with the changes expected of them, and what are the potential financial consequences if they don't? Reimbursement structures are changing, their survival concerns are magnified, and they are bombarded with information about the importance of being patient-centered. They wonder if their perception of being patient-centered is aligned with that of the payer entities that control the practice's financial future. The managed care movement has compromised the trust among patients, physicians, insurance plans, and the healthcare system. How has this cultural shift positioned these key players as they move toward a patient-centered healthcare system?

THE CENTERS FOR MEDICARE & MEDICAID SERVICES (CMS) is putting great emphasis on quality metrics and being *patient-centered*. What this means to physicians, hospitals, and health-care systems around the country is a topic for further discussion and covered in the final chapter of this book. Here we will focus on how we have come to a place where physicians are at odds with healthcare reform and how it might influence the patient-centered movement. We are all aware of the rapid changes going on in the healthcare industry and the physician community. It's a time when physicians cannot stay on the sidelines; instead they need to be an influential partner and central to the solution.

THE CHANGING PHYSICIAN LANDSCAPE

The 2012 Survey of America's Physicians conducted by The Physicians Foundation, in which 13,575 physicians participated, revealed that 43.7% of the respondents were employed physicians.[1] This illustrates a growing trend, with 62% of the physicians under age 40 employed as opposed to 40.2% of the physicians over the age of 40. In this report, Merritt Hawkins revealed that of the 2711 physician-search assignments the firm represented in 2011/2012, less than 1% offered a solo practice, down from 22% percent in 2004.[1] It seems solo physicians are a vanishing breed.

The study further supports the dwindling number of independent physicians as a percentage of total physicians since the year 2000 when 57% of physicians were independent as compared to a projected 33% in 2013.

Physicians are at the vortex of these changes. The way they think, how they are organized, the ways they are evaluated, how they are reimbursed, and their interaction with patients are all subject to partial or complete modification. It is a challenging and uncertain time to be a doctor. The world they live in and the very culture of their profession and their practice are changing.

PHYSICIANS' ATTITUDES TOWARD HEALTHCARE REFORM

Physicians are concerned about the passage of the Patient Protection and Affordable Care Act and its implications: 59% of the survey participants felt less positive about the future of healthcare in America with the passage of this act. Alarmingly, 62% of physicians believed Accountable Care Organizations (ACOs) are unlikely to either increase healthcare quality or decrease costs, indicating that *any quality/cost gains* will not be worth the effort.[1] These attitudes and beliefs are real and reveal a great disparity with organized medicine and the fact that ACOs are being developed at considerable costs and growing rapidly in number at the very same time. This presents a very real conflict. When nearly two thirds of America's physicians have little confidence in the ACO approach, it appears efforts to succeed will be tested, and progress will be somewhat slow.

More than 80% of surveyed physicians believed the medical profession is in decline.

Physicians are also concerned about their income, and for good reason. According to the survey, income was flat for nearly 40% of physicians, and 47% saw their income decline in 2012. And 55% of physicians were unsure about where the American healthcare system will be or how they will fit into it three to five years from now.

These concerns certainly hinder physicians' ability to feel secure about their own future, especially those that are practice owners rather than employees. Physicians have onerous responsibilities that appear to become more burdensome with the expectations of healthcare reform and the quality standards established that affect reimbursement.

The survey also revealed that 58% of the physicians rated their own professional morale as somewhat negative or very negative, and more than 80% believed the medical profession is in decline.[1] The majority of the physicians polled blamed this decline on:

- Too much regulation/paperwork;
- Loss of clinical autonomy;
- Erosion of physician/patient relationship;
- Money trumping patient care; and
- Physicians not compensated for quality.

Some of these findings highlight a stark disparity when compared with the goals of government and organizations that are driving the patient-centered movement. It should be noted that physicians age 39 or younger are less pessimistic about the medical profession with only 16% of these physicians stating that morale was very negative while nearly 25% of those over age 40 felt this way.[1]

PHYSICIANS DESERVE MORE

Delving even further into how physicians feel, when the survey asked, *"Which best describes your attitude toward medical practice today?,"* 41% said "somewhat negative/unsatisfying," while 20% replied "very negative/unsatisfying." Thus 61% of physicians don't feel they are working in a very satisfactory environment, as opposed to the report's findings that less than 34% of the respondents felt that way two years ago (Figure 1).

With America's doctors having little confidence in the ability of ACOs to improve healthcare quality, it seems nearly impossible for doctors to respect the intentions of organized medicine and ACOs. It's as if the leaders and executive teams driving these changes do not value the opinions of physicians. The results of this important study point

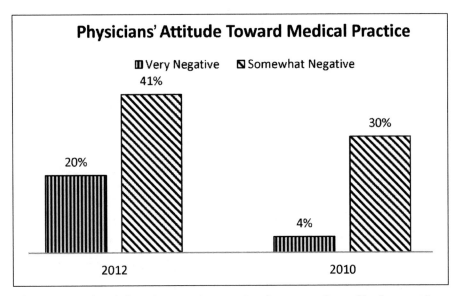

Figure 1. Physicians' negative attitude toward medical practice: 2012 vs. 2010.

to the fact that the voice of America's practicing physicians is not being heard enough, and they have not been engaged by healthcare planners and executives and thus are being left out of the decisions that will change the future of the healthcare delivery system.

To be clear, some physicians in leadership and academic roles have played and will play an important role in the patient-centered movement and the development and intended transformation of the healthcare delivery system; but practicing physicians, as implied in the survey results, are not typically or sufficiently engaged in this effort.

So whether you are a physician, hospital executive, medical practice administrator, or manager, you must wonder how such a movement can succeed with this contrast. It's time for the leaders of the patient-centered movement to engage and communicate better with physicians, listen to their voice, and give them the encouragement and support they need to grow effective partnerships built on trust. If this does not happen, the feelings physicians now share are bound to impede the ability to move swiftly through change and will make the journey to change the cultural mindset of so many physicians far more difficult.

WHAT DRIVES A PATIENT-CENTERED CULTURE?

Physicians may feel they have little influence on the direction of healthcare, but, in fact, they have a great impact on what goes on in their own practice environment. Their attitudes and the relationships they have greatly influence whether or not they create an engaging and positive practice culture that staff members embrace and that is visible to the patients. It is a challenge to accomplish this if they have little confidence in the future of their profession. If physicians believe healthcare reform will bring new opportunities and a future that will improve their existing lack of confidence and plummeting morale and enhance reimbursement, it may have a positive influence on strengthening relationships throughout the industry that will contribute to the greater good.

> *The frequent switching to different physicians in the managed care environment makes it difficult for both patients and physicians to build strong relationships.*

Can physicians and other healthcare providers believe that their concerns are being heard and, more importantly, that the interests of their patients will be protected? This is a tremendous concern at a time when many practicing physicians feel powerless to have influence over the healthcare delivery system, their own future, or the ability to influence the care their patients will receive now and in the future.

RESPECT AND TRUST: CENTRAL TO A CULTURAL SHIFT

Physician Wellness Services and Cejka Search recently completed a nationwide, multispecialty survey of more than 2200 physicians on organizational culture.[2] Of the 14 cultural attributes listed in the survey, the respondents found the following to be of highest priority among physicians:

- Respectful communication;
- Patient-centered care focus and supportive management approach to errors and mistakes; and
- Transparent communication.

Since building and strengthening relationships and overcoming adversity are rooted in mutual respect, one must question how this will be accomplished when the beliefs and attitudes of those that must embrace a culture of change is at odds with the government and industry leaders that are pushing healthcare reform. Physicians seem to have little trust in the motives of government and big insurance companies. They share a deep concern that care will be compromised—not improved—with healthcare reform. "Addressing the physical aspects of patient-centered care is easy," says Susan Frampton, president of Planetree, in Derby, Connecticut. "Changing the culture is difficult to do."[3]

The 2012 Survey of America's Physicians revealed that 38.5% of the physicians believed that hospital employment of physicians will erode the physician/patient relationship and quality of care.[1] This suggests that one third of the physicians have limited confidence in the shifts that are now occurring in the healthcare delivery system, based on healthcare reform initiatives, which will be discussed in the final chapter of this book.

Philosophically, patient-centered care honors the patient and is perceived as the right thing to do. Taking this view, behaviors associated with patient-centered care, such as respecting patients' preferences, should be justified on moral grounds alone, independent of their relationship to health outcomes.[4]

THE PSYCHOLOGY OF THE CONSUMER

Everyone wants to be respected, and the patient-centered movement is aimed at ensuring patients are respected, understand their choices, and are more involved in their own healthcare decisions. A 2005 Johns Hopkins study of 5514 American consumers examined the issue of respect. The study revealed that patients who said they were treated with respect during their last medical experience were likely to be more satisfied and adhere more closely to therapy than those that were not.[5] This certainly suggests that respecting patients results in more compliant patients. It seems physicians are on the right track with respecting patients since 76% of those surveyed said they were treated with a great deal of respect during their last medical encounter.[5]

ONCE UPON A TIME

Years ago, patients would choose a physician and remain with that physician for many years, making a change only if they moved or their healthcare condition required more specialized care. There was loyalty and a strong bond between the physician and the patient. Physicians knew their patients' families, and patients had tremendous trust in and respect for physicians. It was a time when physicians referred back and forth between specialties without concern for patients' healthcare insurance, and patients had confidence they were always getting the best of care, just ask anyone that's a baby boomer or older. Anyone younger would be unlikely to recall such a time, as they grew up in the managed care era where insurance companies have limited patients' choices and often dictate the physicians they select and the care they get.

This is not to suggest the world of medicine was great and patients had no complaints. At that time, medical practices were run by physicians with little or no training about business. They had little understanding of operational efficiency or the staffing skills and experience required to run a prudent business. Their office manager was often someone that came up through the ranks that was hard-working and dependable, but lacked formal business education having learned on the job most of what he or she knew about a medical practice. In fact, some physicians still select staff members without placing enough value on business education. Physicians were able to make independent decisions on how they practiced and cared for patients, and life was easier for them. Because doctors set their charges and were paid accordingly with few exceptions, they always made a good living and were financially secure, whether the practice was well-run or not. Yet even in those good old days, the reception room was often packed with waiting patients and standing room only. No, practicing medicine and patient service were not perfect, but much of the time physicians had far more independence, and patients could make their own healthcare decisions.

THE IMPACT OF MANAGED CARE

Since the emergence of managed care in the late 1980s and its national explosion in the 1990s, employers shift insurance plans frequently, sometimes annually, in their attempts to contain the costs of healthcare benefits they offer their employees. Patients, in an effort to have lower insurance costs, often pick the low-cost option the employer offers. This results in patients changing their insurance plans frequently. Since each insurance plan has its own physician panel, based on those medical practices willing to sign a contract at the reimbursement and terms offered by the plan, this sometimes means patients must switch to another primary care physician (PCP). Patients can usually stay with their physician if the doctor is not contracted with their new insurance plan, but at a greater out-of-pocket cost for the patient that stings family finances. It is a financial choice, but most patients move on—letting the insurance plan dictate their choices.

> ### The patient-centered movement is aimed at ensuring patients are respected.

Managed care changed the rules of healthcare delivery. For over 15 years, healthcare providers have struggled with the lower, stagnant reimbursement and diminished control of patient care brought about by managed care. This has resulted in a change in physicians' attitude about how they work and the attention patients get, thereby eroding the patient experience. Hospitals facing the financial challenges of managed care have similar struggles in their attempts to contain costs. Patients complain that a visit to the emergency department can be a nightmare, and patients are often discharged from the hospital based on their insurance plan's limitation, even though they aren't confident their condition has improved enough to be managed at home. This leaves some of them feeling abandoned and worried that their healthcare is being compromised. It's hard for patients to believe the hospital has their best interest at heart in these types of situations, yet the hospital can feel hamstrung because of the limitations on what the insurance plan will pay it.

It's a challenge for both the hospital and the physician that discharges the patient, who could well be a hospitalist physician employed by the hospital. This can create a *disconnect* for the patient and the PCP that will manage the after-discharge care. If the communication and coordination does not go well, the patient feels vulnerable, and the PCP feels frustrated and helpless.

Dealing with the insurance company is another matter. Patients may have to accept the limitations of their insurance plan, but that doesn't mean they have to like it! Trying to reach someone that has answers, a vested interest in helping, or any power in the customer service department of the insurance company is nearly impossible. Patients complain when insurance companies control where they go and what tests they receive, and are more than a little annoyed when these types of things delay treatment.

THE PHYSICIAN-PATIENT RELATIONSHIP SUFFERS

The frequent switching to different physicians in the managed care environment makes it difficult for both patients and physicians to build strong relationships. It can also compromise the continuity and coordination of care. It is frustrating for both patients and physicians. Physicians are less satisfied, sometimes feeling that on top of reduced reimbursement they no longer have control over their own patients' care. They also see a decline in the respect they get from patients and sometimes feel like their practice has become a turnstile of patients, some of them more demanding and far less trusting than in the pre-managed care days.

In stressed or unmotivated practices, patients may feel the doctor doesn't know anything personal about them or their family or even care much, even if the entire family goes to the same medical practice. Sometimes staff members show zero interest in the patients and are perfunctory in performing their tasks during the patients' office visit. No one seems to smile, including the patients. Patients don't feel they really get to know their doctor and are quite sure the physician doesn't remember anything much about them. They aren't impressed with the service they get whether they stay with one practice or switch to another.

Patients don't like this, but they have learned to accept less from their healthcare experiences. They can have trouble getting an appointment at a medical facility too busy to care. When they do, they often enter a facility that hasn't been updated in years, are greeted by sullen staff, and have to wait 30 or 40 minutes to see their healthcare provider.

Not only is access for an appointment poor, but try to get through to your physician, diagnostic center, or allied treatment facility on the phone. The patient will either wait on hold for an unreasonable period of time; be jockeyed around among employees trying to get help; or find that the phones are shut down for the first hour of the morning, during a two-hour lunch break, and by 5:00 PM. It's an impossible situation. All these things exist in so many healthcare facilities, both large and small, that it seems to be the acceptable standard of care. It's not a pretty picture, but many patients have just learned to accept it—until now that is.

PATIENTS FINALLY SPEAK OUT

Patients have been empowered by the Internet and are speaking their piece, as explained in detail in Chapter 4. They are going online and rating the physician experience for the entire world to see. Even though this is not a scientific, objective approach to rating doctors and staff, it seems legitimate and has the power to influence the reader that is searching online to find out more about a healthcare provider or facility. In addition, the patient-centered movement has resulted in patients being surveyed by lots of different entities: private insurance plans, hospitals, Medicare, health systems, and even some employers. Unfortunately, as stated in Chapter 1, patients' bias and emotional response to some surveys can create skewed results and place undue pressure on physicians to appease patients in order to achieve good scores.

Consumerism is pushing doctors to deliver patient-centered care. It has been prevalent in other industries for centuries, but now it is a force in the healthcare delivery system. "Consumer-driven health-care, a new benefits strategy, is poised to change the way healthcare consumers make decisions," according to Jeff Ozmon, MBA. "The most dramatic changes will occur in the primary care setting, where consumers seeking routine care traditionally have paid only relatively small co-payments. With health savings plans and high-deductible insurance plans, consumers seeking routine medical care will now be responsible for the entire first dollar charge up to the required deductible."[6] This will likely result in many patients being more discerning healthcare shoppers and giving them a more influential voice in matters involving their healthcare.

THE JOURNEY CONTINUES

We believe the journey is long and worthy, and the leaders of the patient-centered movement are well-intended. If the cultural differences and what it takes to change the culture are recognized and respected, progress will continue. And if physician trust and confidence in the healthcare system and its leaders can be restored, essential partnerships among key stakeholders will grow and be strengthened.

Consumerism is pushing doctors to deliver patient-centered care.

Transforming patient care to a more patient-centered system will require working together in a collaborative, interdependent system and in forming a true partnership between the healthcare system and the people it serves. The actions taken by healthcare leaders will influence at what rate this shift occurs and how quickly the desired goals of a patient-centered healthcare system are achieved. This is an ambitious movement, and the journey continues.

THE PAYOFF

If healthcare planners and executives succeed in engaging America's practicing physicians by giving them a voice to weigh-in on the future of healthcare, these leaders can impact physicians' understanding of healthcare reform and the opportunities it offers. This will strengthen relationships within the industry, contributing to success for providers and patients alike in a patient-centered future.

References

1. Merritt Hawkins. A Survey of America's Physicians: Practice Patterns and Perspectives. The Physicians Foundation. September 2012; www.physiciansfoundation.org/health-care-research/a-survey-of-americas-physicians-practice-patterns-and-perspectives/.
2. Stark R. Organizational culture: addressing satisfaction gaps around cultural fit. *Physician Magazine*. May 2013:10.
3. Defining, Measuring and Sustaining a Patient-Centered Culture. Planetree. http://planetreegrove.com/wp-content/uploads/2013/01/Defining-measuring-and-sustaining-a-patient-centered-culture.pdf.
4. Epstein RM, Street RL Jr. The values and value of patient-centered care. *Ann Fam Med*. 2011;9(2):100-103.
5. Johns Hopkins Medical Institutions. Patients Treated With Respect More Likely to Follow Medical Advice. September 1, 2005; www.hopkinsmedicine.org/Press_releases/2005/08_31b_05.html.
6. Ozmon J. Consumerism: forcing medical practice toward patient-centered care. *J Med Pract Manage*. 2007;23:44-46.

CHAPTER 8

Mirror, Mirror: An Honest Look Within

To meet your organization's full potential for success, you must look honestly at the experience you provide to patients. And even with your best efforts, it can prove extremely difficult, if not impossible, to do so objectively because you never *will be* your patient. Through years of interviewing patients, conducting hundreds of surveys, making mystery patient visits, and partnering with practices to improve their patients' experience, we have gained insight into the psychology of patients that proves to be a powerful tool for success when properly applied.

I N CHAPTER 1, we talked about how consultants are often called into medical practices, hospitals, and other healthcare organizations (both large and small) to address stagnant or declining revenue, staffing issues, and workflow efficiency, but rarely for the purpose of improving the patient experience. Why? There are a few reasons; one being that the natural bias and desire to assume the best of our own performance can blind us to needed change. Another reason is fear. Most small businesses avoid providing customers with avenues to give honest feedback out of a fear that they will hear something that is painful, embarrassing, or difficult to repair.

There is also a lack of understanding of how connected patient satisfaction is to the overall success of a practice. A fresh focus on the patient experience can often contribute to resolving other issues and bring improvements that lead to greater success. When leaders communicate a fearless and no-blame attitude—and explain that they themselves are being rated and taking an honest look at their *own* performance—then patient feedback can be embraced by staff as a catalyst to an improved patient experience and increased job fulfillment as the practice thrives.

Research indicates that for every complaint expressed there are more than 25 unregistered complaints.[1] That means that for every unhappy patient you hear from or are aware of, there are likely another twenty-something experiencing the same dissatisfaction that opt to remain silent. When considering how infrequently a patient with a less-than-satisfactory experience will speak up and tell you the source of his or her angst, it's easy to see how false assumptions of patient satisfaction can be made. Taking an honest look at the patient experience you provide is not just brave and important, it's crucial to reaping the high ratings, loyal patients, referrals, and stellar online reputation that practices that are among the best aim for.

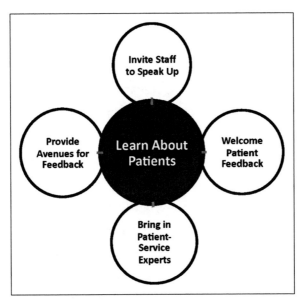

FIGURE 1. Learn more about your patients.

STAND ABOVE THE REST

We all love to hear that we're doing a great job, but those practices that stand head and shoulders above the rest are the ones that are willing to take an honest look in the mirror and embrace a culture of constant improvement based on professional assessments and patient feedback (Figure 1). Here are four ways a practice, ambulatory surgery center, or hospital can begin to better understand its patients' perspective and the experience being provided to patients, and identify opportunities to improve:

1. **Invite staff to speak up.** Gather your staff together to communicate your intent to better understand the needs and desires of patients and make changes to meet those needs. Communicate to your staff members that complaints should be viewed as opportunities to improve, and you want everyone to share what they are hearing from patients without fear that those comments will reflect poorly on staff performance.

2. **Provide anonymous avenues for patients.** Just as statistics show that customers are more likely to quietly take their business elsewhere than they are to complain, so it is with patients. They may fear a negative remark will affect future care they receive or reflect poorly on them. They may think it's not worth the hassle because it won't change anything. Providing anonymous forms of surveying will result in more honest, and more helpful, feedback. Make it as easy as possible for patients to speak up: send an e-mail survey via a service like Constant Contact or Survey Monkey, provide point-of-service comment cards that are dropped in a box anonymously, or simply ask in person, "Is there anything we can do to improve your experience at our practice?" Then actually track those comments and bring them to decision-makers. When surveying, make it short and simple, and always leave space for comments.

3. **Communicate your culture of welcoming feedback.** We've all been in a store, restaurant, or other business that provided poor service yet offered a comment card. You wonder if filling it out would make any difference, and likely decide not to waste your time. In a practice where patient feedback is valued and welcomed, this message must be communicated verbally and in the survey tool itself. Remember, the most effective way to communicate your commitment is by responding to the feedback with improvements. Its okay to "toot your own horn" by announcing, "We heard you, and we are making this change based on our patients' feedback." To patients, that translates into: "We *really do* care about you, we *really are* committed to winning your loyalty, and you're getting top-notch care here."

4. **Call in the experts.** Patients and staff members will provide you with great feedback and internal, hands-on ideas for improvement, but there is a time and place to call in experts who have a greater understanding of possible offerings and solutions.

Mystery patient services, for example, are conducted by experts qualified to look for certain criteria that patients and staff may not know how to verbalize or recognize. Another way experts can help you uncover great opportunities for improvement and the deeper needs or desires of patients is by conducting third-party interviews and surveys. Patients are more honest and open with a third party because they don't feel self conscience about the staff knowing "who said what."

Quantitative feedback is obtained through large-scale surveys from which patterns can be detected and bulk information analyzed. On the other hand, third-party interviews with patients result in *qualitative feedback* that provides deeper insight as patients are given a platform to share openly and are probed further about specific issues.

When considering changes that could impact the patient experience such as adding a new service line, providing alternative clinic hours, or changing a billing policy, a professional can successfully extract honest feedback from a focus group of patients, analyze the data, and report on findings that can save your organization significant time, money, and effort by avoiding a bad decision or implementing a welcome change in a specific way.

UNDERSTANDING PATIENTS

There are certain truths that apply to patients regardless of what kind of practice, clinic, or health organization you are part of. Understanding the psychology of patients can equip physicians, practice leaders, and staff members to empathize with and meet the needs of patients with improved education, communication, and sincerity.

It sounds so obvious, but sometimes those working in healthcare need reminding that patients are not where they want to be when they are visiting you. It's usually not a good day if they are ill or receiving treatment. Perhaps they are about to have a screening that you've been performing all day, every day for 12 years. But it's their first one—*ever*. And they are so afraid they couldn't sleep the night before. A flippant, casual attitude is going to come off as unprofessional, uncompassionate, and detached.

A lackadaisical attitude toward a patient's healthcare will communicate that staff members don't really care to understand what patients are feeling or meet their emotional needs in regard to their visit. In this situation, do you think patients will struggle with changing providers should they have even the slightest reason to switch? Nope. It's easy to lose sight of this, but it's imperative to understanding patients' needs. Patients usually have more on their minds than what they communicate to you directly. It may not show on the outside but patients have fears and worry about:

- **Money.** How much is this going to cost me? Can I afford it? Will it lead to more expense? Will I miss work and lose pay? Will I have to buy expensive prescriptions? And for caretakers: Will I be out of work to take care of my parent, child, or spouse because of this health issue? Can my loved one afford this care, or will I be responsible?
- **Pain.** Will this hurt? How long will it hurt? Will it lead to more procedures or complications that hurt? Will I have to take pain medication? And for caretakers: Is my loved one going to be in pain, which causes us both emotional stress?
- **Time.** How long will this take? Will I make it to my next appointment, childcare pick-up, or shift? Will I be laid up afterward? Who will have time to care of me, my kids, my parent, my home if I can't? And for caretakers: How will I find the time to care for my loved one with all my other responsibilities?

Understanding patients better will help you know how to meet their needs; and in return, you will have happier, calmer, and more compliant patients who are ready to listen because their fears have been eased. It will actually make everyone's job easier. Every practice is unique in how it will address its patients' concerns about money, pain, and time—but be sure you do address them. Assure patients, answer their questions in full, educate them up front, offer a word of comfort, and ask them to tell you what they need.

Patients will often reveal what they need to hear when they sense a staff member is tuned into them. When a patient arrives for a visit and realizes she will be seeing a doctor she hasn't seen before and tentatively says, "Oh . . . I've never met Dr. Newbie before . . . ," a staff reply of, "Dr. Newbie has been in his field for seven years, and our other patients love him; you are in good hands" can make all the difference. The odds that Dr. Newbie will enter the exam room to find a receptive, more relaxed patient have just improved significantly as does the patient's confidence in the physician, the patient experience, and the image of a cohesive practice. Front-line staff members can be trained to respond to these cues effectively, contributing to a patient experience that benefits the entire practice while gaining a sense of pride in the value they bring to the practice and patients.

THE POWER OF LISTENING

It may take a minute longer, but making sure you hear what patients are trying to communicate pays off. You will respond more accurately with what they *really* want to know, which will improve cooperation and compliance, prevent the need for a call to the office later for clarification, and increase patients' sense of being valued, which is directly related to increased patient satisfaction scores.[2]

Active listening requires that the listener gain clarification by paraphrasing back to the speaker the idea that's just been communicated. In doing this, the speaker gains a sense of being heard as well as an opportunity to correct the listener if he or she hasn't gotten it right. It doesn't take a lot of time and can result in a far more meaningful,

Tips for Successful Communication with Patients

1. Assure patients that you are listening by:
   a. Repeating back in paraphrases, "So after the fever subsided, you experienced a dry cough for two weeks and then the fever returned?"
   b. Facing the patient with your entire body and making eye contact whenever possible.
   c. Displaying empathy by saying things like, "I'm sorry you've been unable to sleep, let's see what we can do to get you a good night's rest again" or by a concerned facial expression.
   d. Giving an occasional nod or leaning in and saying, "Uh-huh."
2. Ask for questions. You will be surprised how much more you find out when you signal to your patient that you are interested in the full picture by asking questions like, "Is there anything else you want to address today?" and "Do you have any questions?" This seemingly small step is very significant to patients and contributes to increased patient satisfaction and participation, while giving you important additional information.
3. Stand, or sit, eye to eye. When one person stands over or above another while communicating, it can imply superiority. Whenever possible, communicate at the same eye level to imply equality and partnership.
4. Talk through your actions. Communicating what you are about to do or why you are doing something is a great way to honor patients and

effective patient visit. In giving this feedback, clinicians and staff may find that an assumption they made is incorrect, and this could change the diagnosis and treatment recommendation. It's important, however, to remember that jumping in to reiterate too soon—before the patient is done speaking—can give the impression that you want to rush the patient out the door. The importance of ensuring that patients are given ample time to communicate is demonstrated in these statistics:

- In 37% of primary care visits, physicians ask patients about the reason for their visit, but interrupt the patients after hearing express concern for their well-being. Some examples are, "I'd like to examine your spine now, so would you turn around and bend over?," "I'm using this hand gel to protect you," and "I'm pulling this curtain to give you privacy." Letting patients know what's coming next, asking for their consent, and letting them know the reason for the things you are doing give patients a much-needed sense of control over a situation they may be fearful of.

5. Pay attention to body language. In the midst of considering the health history and listening to your patient, you might not consider what they are *not* verbalizing. Body language accounts for 55% of communication, and tone of voice accounts for 38%—leaving just 7% for actual words.[3] That means you could pick up on more clues by watching your patients' gestures and tone of voice. Likewise, you can send the wrong message if your arms are crossed, you don't make eye contact, or your hand is on the doorknob as you speak (indicating the patient is holding you back from where you really want to go).

6. Use the patient's name. This simple addition to a sentence makes a big impact, especially when repeated throughout the visit. Phrases such as, "Thank you, Mr. Sage," "Johanna, are you comfortable with taking a sleeping aid?" and "I'm sorry to hear you've been in pain, Josh" are just another way to shout, "You're important here, and we know you." And really, that's exactly what patients want to hear.

the first concern mentioned and proceed to the history and physical exam.[4]

- When taking a medical history, physicians collect only 60% of essential history items from patients.[5]
- Fifty percent of patients typically report having "unvoiced concerns" at the end of the visit.[6]

In the business office of your practice and throughout your organization, improved communication can reduce frustration between staff and patients by clarifying intentions. For example, suppose a patient is asked for payment for her child's visit before being seen, and she tells the staff that she isn't able to pay until later. The staff member politely asks when she will be able to pay, and finds out that she intends to pay on the way out because her husband will be meeting her there and he has the checkbook. If instead of asking the patient about paying, the staff member had sternly stated that payment before the visit is the practice policy and the visit cannot take place until payment has been received, the patient would have been misunderstood and felt devalued, possibly even embarrassed and angry.

> *A fresh focus on the patient experience can often contribute to resolving other issues and bring improvements that lead to greater success.*

In a clinical setting, reiterating back to patients what they are experiencing and reporting as far as symptoms and duration is not just important for the obvious reasons of improved accuracy, it also assures patients they are being heard and valued, thus improving their satisfaction and compliance. In a survey of more than 2300 adults in the United States, 71% said it was more important that they connect with their doctor personally than to have a doctor with top credentials.[7]

RESEARCH SPOTLIGHTS COMMUNICATION

According to research presented in *Mayo Clinic Proceedings*, seven "ideal physician behaviors" were identified from patient interviews. Patients in the study wanted their physicians to be "confident, empathetic, humane, personal, forthright, respectful and thorough."[8] Most of the communication skills above involve at least two or three of these attributes.

While communication has long been thought of as a "soft" science, it's increasingly being understood to be at the root of many of healthcare's biggest shortfalls and a leading culprit in rising costs. Research shows that when physicians don't listen to patients, they can miss important health cues and misdiagnose illnesses. Patients who don't fully understand what their doctors say fail to follow their treatment regimens, which can lead to preventable hospitalizations, complications, and poor outcomes. "If patients don't understand their discharge instructions, they are less likely to be compliant and more likely to be readmitted, so it is critically important that everyone uses effective communication tools and language," says Christina Martin, director of service coaching and patient experience at WellStar Health System, based in Marietta, Georgia.[9]

If this isn't compelling enough to inspire you to take a hard look at communication in your organization, consider the legal implications of poor communication in healthcare. A breakdown in physician-patient communication is cited in 40% or more of malpractice suits. However, "If a doctor and patient have a strong relationship, even if something goes wrong, they are less likely to sue for it," says Robin Diamond, chief patient safety officer at Doctors Co., which provides malpractice insurance for 73,000 physicians and holds communication seminars.[10] Taking the time and effort to communicate clearly, compassionately, and thoroughly helps build the team mentality needed for successful healthcare outcomes.

CASE STUDY

TMI (Too Much Information): Thanks but No Thanks!

We've all encountered "too much of a good thing." The same holds true when communicating with patients. Just as it's important to keep in mind that your patients aren't familiar with the specialty and procedures of your practice, it's important to know that they might *not want* to know all the clinical details. Here is an example of a patient who found herself getting an education she didn't ask for.

Sophie Winters was referred to oral surgeon Jose Carlos, DDS, by her dentist. Dr. Carlos was friendly, informative, and confident. Sophie was being seen for excessive gum recession; and sure enough, Dr. Carlos felt a gum graft was in order. Sophie was expecting this and though she was a bit nervous, she was ready to schedule the procedure. But Dr. Carlos assumed she would want to know more about the procedure. Not wanting to offend him, Sophie acted interested and even asked questions as she found herself naturally curious. She thought, "Wow, he's willing to spend this extra time with me, I should oblige." At the same time, her apprehension increased as Dr. Carlos showed her computerized images of how a gum graft is performed. Of course, she knew it was important for her to understand that the graft would come from the roof of her mouth and be placed where the recession was worst. But even so, seeing it all play out on a video on Dr. Carlos' laptop was not easing her fears. Dr. Carlos went on and on, using medical terms and going into great detail. She found herself completely lost and thinking about other things. The doctor was friendly and enthusiastic—eager to share a field he studied and had a passion for. Unfortunately, Sophie left feeling more apprehensive and over-educated in what she didn't really need or want to know.

When surgery day came, she was nervous, but ready. She opted to not be put "under" as she'd never had trouble with having fillings or crowns, and she figured as long as she didn't feel anything, she could do this. This can-do attitude slowly but surely left her over the next two hours. The entire procedure took far longer than expected, she heard sounds of cutting and felt tugging, her mouth was open for two hours, and she began to panic. There was nothing she could do, they were halfway through the procedure already, and she found herself holding back tears and resisting the urge to flee. Through self-talk and breathing techniques she'd learned in preparation for childbirth, she was able to make it through what was a very traumatic experience for her.

Sophie had been over-educated in what she neither wanted nor needed to know, and yet was totally unprepared for the experience of the procedure. She was uninformed of the length of time the procedure would take and how much further up the psychological tolerance ladder this was from a filling or crown. She was shocked at how long the recovery took, and how painful it was to eat and even drink. Dr. Carlos was doing so many things right—he was friendly, confident, willing to spend time communicating with his patient—and yet he missed the mark. Surely, Dr. Carlos assumed Sophie was well prepared after his lengthy explanation of the procedure. Without systems in place to obtain honest feedback from patients, physicians and staff make these kinds of assumptions over and over without ever knowing—and it's costly in so many ways.

NAVIGATING A FINE LINE

Take cues from patients, and give them the basic information of why, what, and who. Educate your patients in why something is recommended, what can or will be done, and who will do it. This is a good time to boost patients' confidence by letting them know this person is, "referred to all the time for this procedure" or "has done over 400 of these procedures without complications." Then ask if they have questions or want resources to learn more about how the procedure or treatment works. Telling patients the risks, especially if there are specific or additional risks for their situation (i.e., due to being overweight or another condition), is essential communication, but the amount of detail you provide on how a procedure is performed can be simplified for patients who would rather trust you to do your job, and leave it at that.

The important thing to remember is that for you *and* those patients who don't want TMI, a simple explanation of *why, what,* and *who* is efficient and sufficient. Many larger practices, hospitals, and health systems are equipped with allied support staff, such as a nurse educator or patient coordinator, trained to provide this information in terms that are easily understood and accepted by patients. Offering to go further to answer questions if they want more information—and pointing them to your Web site or other reputable resources for additional information—is usually enough to satisfy everyone.

IT REALLY *IS* ALL ABOUT THEM

Most patients don't work in the field of healthcare, so they aren't familiar with the terminology of your practice or even general healthcare terms having to do with billing and insurance. Staff members that are on the front line must learn to use pedestrian terminology, simplifying the process for patients whenever possible. Remember the worries on patients' minds: money, pain, and time? In addition, patients are trying to memorize what the doctor says to them. Add insurance-speak or overly clinical terms to the mix, and you're sure to have patients with mounting frustration. Asking a patient, "Who told you that?" when no one in your practice wears a name badge may cause the patient to feel stupid and powerless. What seems obvious to staff is not always obvious to patients. They can't differentiate between credentials, and often assume anyone in scrubs is clinically trained staff.

Make it as easy as possible for patients to speak up.

Name badges with credentials are important in empowering patients as well as a legal requirement in some states. For instance, in Illinois, the state's Medical Patient Rights Act requires licensed healthcare facility employees, including students, and volunteers who examine or treat patients to wear an identification badge stating their first name, licensure status, and staff position.[11] A strict protocol that all staff members wear identification that is legible for all patients (including older, vision-impaired patients) is a fantastic way to empower patients, improve communication, and present an overall image of professionalism, accountability, and pride.

WHAT YOU CAN DO NOW

It isn't easy to look at things from the other side of the stethoscope or check-in desk, but the fact that you are reading this book means you know it's important and you want to succeed. Though we recommend obtaining mystery patient services and having your facility professionally assessed, there is something you can do immediately that will cost very little and could provide valuable insight: conduct your own study.

Either you or a designated staff member who is a customer service champion and fearless in giving feedback will be given the day or half day to investigate the practice from the patients' perspective. That means you will park where patients park when they have to vie for spots (not before hours when the lot is empty). Imagine that you don't know where the office is; are there signs pointing you in the right direction? What was your experience getting from your car to the office? Consider your patient base, do they use strollers or walkers?

Walk in the same door that patients use to see and experience the practice as they do. Sit in the reception area, listen to the communication between the front desk and patients, and spend time observing in each area. Ask permission of patients to observe the examination, and conduct a brief interview afterward asking if there is anything the practice or facility can do to improve their experience.

Are you required to sign your name on a sign-in sheet where other patients could see it? Were the magazines old and the carpet dirty? Could you overhear preoperative instructions for another patient? Did the receptionist announce why someone was there so that the entire reception room heard it?

You won't see things the same way as an objective, trained expert who has specific criteria to look for and the benefit of an unbiased viewpoint, but you may still come up with some great new ideas to improve the patient experience!

CASE STUDY
From Unsettling to Soothing

In one mystery patient visit, we found a framed antique black-and-white photo of a row of surgeons from the late 1800s or early 1900s dressed in gloves and masks, standing in front of an operating table and what is now antiquated equipment. The photo conjured up feelings of "old medicine"—you know, the days when they gave you a bullet to bite as they sawed off your leg. The kicker is that the photo was hanging in the procedure room of the practice—where patients would be feeling most vulnerable and fearful.

This open-minded physician came to understand how patients might not view and appreciate the photo the way he did. Needless to say, the photo was replaced. Instead of an image that could provoke fear, a large picture of a tranquil beach was hung. This was strategically placed where it could be viewed by patients from the procedure table, providing a visual escape. The original picture is surely still enjoyed by the physician, but now is out of the view of patients. With regard for the client's appreciation of photography and the practice's coastal location, the replacement is a black-and-white photo of a beach with soft rolling waves with hints of color artistically added. Even the most enthusiastic, well-meaning staff and physicians can be oblivious to the patients' perspective at times.

CONSIDER YOUR PATIENT DEMOGRAPHICS

Top-notch practices and hospitals get to know the needs of their patients and meet them—not just the patients' health needs, but understanding the small nuances so that service is provided in a way that fits the patients' lifestyle. Practices that provide elective services and compete for dollars from patients outside of insurance plans have embraced this kind of patient courting in order to survive, but any healthcare system can boost its competitive edge and promote loyalty by taking a deeper look at the practical needs and lifestyle of its target patients.

> *Patients usually have more on their minds than what they communicate to you directly.*

What do we mean by demographics and lifestyle? We mean considering the lifestyle needs of the patients you want to attract or that make up the bread and butter of your patient mix. Let's consider, for example, a practice or department of a health system that sees geriatric patients. Considering the needs of this type of patient is extremely important in shaping the patient experience. For example, parking should be adjacent or as close as possible to where patients will be seen. The walk to the office should not require patients to take stairs or involve risky or narrow paths that inhibit the use of walkers or require patients to open heavy doors. For this demographic, forms should be provided in large print, and unnecessary noise or music that makes it difficult to hear should be eliminated or reduced whenever possible. Communication should be particularly slow and clear about issues that may cause confusion or anxiety such as payment, the content of forms the patients are asked to sign, directions for aftercare, or referrals. And chairs need to have arms on them, giving older patients a way to push themselves up to standing.

Or if your practice sees teens that are racing in after school or between extracurricular activities, find out if providing workspace for doing homework makes sense. It did in an orthodontist's office we visited. However, a water feature in an OB/GYN's office, though pretty, might not be welcomed by women who already find themselves in the restroom more often then they'd like.

A Shopper's Anecdote
by Coauthor Cheryl Bisera

There is a particular department store where I like to shop; it carries clothing for women and teens in adjoining departments. That means I can shop for my daughter and myself at the same time, I can look in both departments for either of us because they merge, and I like the quality and price point. However, the music is geared to teens. That means I, and all the other women, have to listen to wailing electric guitars and questionable lyrics during our "me time." That doesn't work for me—and I am the one with the wallet. It's downright irritating most of the time, and I don't stay long. Recently, I popped in to look for a specific item for my daughter, and I noticed the music had changed. It was in the middle—something I could enjoy without being too "old school" for teens. Looks like someone got the message. Catering to the specific needs of patients makes *your brand's* healthcare fit *their* lifestyle, and you will reap the benefits of referrals when they talk to friends and family about the convenience and perks that differentiate you.

Look at the statistics of your patient base, and consider what their lives look like. Can the over-50 crowd read the light-colored or small font on your Web site? Do after-hours commuters get a bottle of water and a granola bar as they wait to be seen after a long day at work? Can you make appointments feel more like "me time" for early-morning physical therapy patients by providing a coffee station?

BOOKS *ARE* JUDGED BY THEIR COVER: STAFF APPEARANCE

Think of members of your entire staff as ambassadors of your brand; they represent your facility, your hospital, your physicians—perhaps a practice that someone spent years dreaming of, studying for, and planning for in order to realize his or her dream of opening a private practice. I think that's worth considering when setting standards. Just as clinical errors can take down a practice and destroy a reputation, staff image and presentation can do the same, albeit slowly and quietly.

No, having a brash receptionist dressed in spiked leather may not land you in a scandalous front-page exposé, but it does chip away at the professional image and confidence you want to instill in patients. People are people. We can't please them all, and it's a delicate balance of not overreaching with employees. So how do you tackle this seemingly subjective topic without making enemies?

First of all, it's important that organizations implement a dress code early on. Don't wait until there is a problem to formulate your standards. Addressing this issue in any way other than objectively, specifically, and by protocol can stir up division, resentment, offense, and even accusations of discrimination. So take the bull by the horns, and write a concise dress code that addresses even the minute details (think worst-case scenario) of what is and is not acceptable for your brand representatives—your staff. All things considered, not every healthcare organization or practice needs to have the same guidelines. Your patient demographic, specialty, and even geographic location can all come into play. However, a professional and cohesive image should be at the heart of every dress code policy (Figure 2).

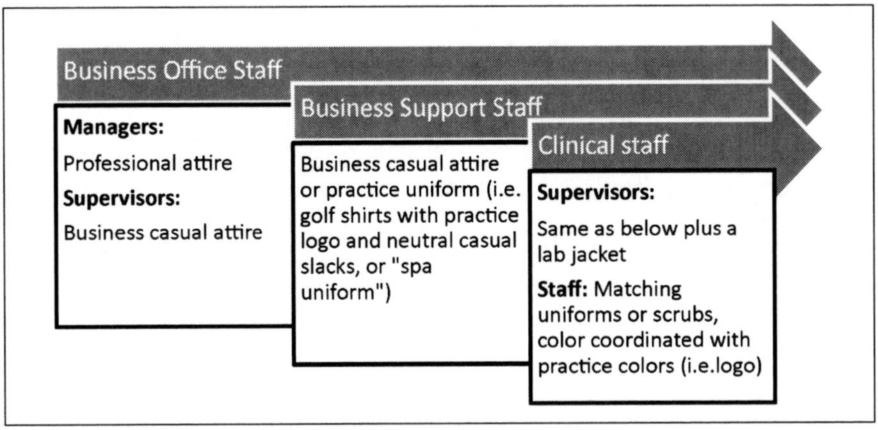

Business Office Staff

Managers:
Professional attire

Supervisors:
Business casual attire

Business Support Staff

Business casual attire or practice uniform (i.e. golf shirts with practice logo and neutral casual slacks, or "spa uniform")

Clinical staff

Supervisors:
Same as below plus a lab jacket

Staff: Matching uniforms or scrubs, color coordinated with practice colors (i.e.logo)

FIGURE 2. Exploring staff attire.

Your staff members represent a professional healthcare team to your patients. They represent your values, commitment, clinical training, overall brand, and competence. It's important that they look like the team your patients would choose to handle one of the most important areas of their lives! Yet how often do we walk into a practice to find both office and clinical staff wearing baggy, drawstring scrubs in mix-and-match styles and colors? Why is it that bank tellers who handle our money are required to look professional, and those assisting in our healthcare (also very important to us) look like they are in their pajamas? What message do we send when staff comfort and laziness takes precedence over professional appearance? Think about your sick patients who get themselves up and dressed to come obtain care from you. They have an excuse to be lazy and comfortable. They often feel horrible, but they value how they present themselves, and they respect the nature of their visit. Healthcare workers should look professional. Why are we picking on you? You may feel your heart rate rising because you feel we are being unfair and unreasonable . . . perhaps even disrespectful. We *are* talking straight here, but there is no disrespect. In fact, we respect your position, the influence you have on the patient experience, and the image of the practice or brand you represent so much that we believe your attire should match the professionalism and importance of that position.

Take a moment to consider the brand of your practice, clinic, or hospital. Is the brand and its values communicated in the most professional way by the appearance of its staff representatives? If scrubs are determined to be the best choice for clinical staff, do they match? Are they color coordinated to reinforce the brand? Is there uniformity to communicate a cohesive team and pride? Does the color of staff uniforms resemble something unsettling to patients— like black, which can be associated with death, or red, which can be associated with blood? Again, keeping in mind patients' fears, worries, and concerns will help guide these decisions.

Are nonclinical staff dressed professionally? One must question if it makes sense for front office or billing staff to wear scrubs. These nonclinical positions represent the patient service and business ambassadors of the practice. Remember the bank teller. Most likely a uniform or professional dress code would be a better choice for these key players—but don't forget the name badge *and the smile!*

We've worked with practices desiring to build up the elective procedure portion of their service mix. One way to do this is to give patients a more lavish, spa-like experience while maintaining a professional medical atmosphere. Dressing staff to look the part can be accomplished with uniforms that go beyond scrubs. With a simple online search under "spa uniforms," you can find uniform retailers like Noel Asmar Uniforms (noelasmaruniforms.com) that provide flattering, tailored options that are a few notches above scrubs yet comfortable and flattering.

> *The most effective way to communicate your commitment is by responding to patient feedback with improvements.*

One of our clients, Peterson Pierre, MD, a cosmetic dermatologist and founder of Pierre Skin Care Institute, took this idea to the next level by providing his staff with a winter/fall color and a spring/summer color set of uniforms. His employees love the durable, flattering uniforms that save them money and time in the mornings—as well as having a change of color halfway through the year.

Another suggestion is to have staff wear matching polo shirts in one of the practice colors and khaki or grey pants. If Target can do this—and we all know to look for someone in a red top and khaki bottoms when we need help while shopping there—so can the healthcare industry. Sometimes it's wise to take a lesson from nonhealth-related businesses that are leaders in customer satisfaction, confidence, and loyalty. Patients want to feel satisfied, confident, and loyal toward their healthcare providers—help them along and reap the rewards!

Dress Code Standards

Your standards and values *will* be communicated, at least somewhat, through your staff's appearance. For this reason, it is pertinent to think through what you really don't want patients to see, and have it in writing, with each new employee signing an agreement to comply, *before* you have a problem. Be specific. If a ring on each finger is too many, say so. If you don't want tattoos to be visible or perfumes to be detectable, say so. Blue hair? You bet you should cover it! If you can dream it, it can happen. But remember, if you aren't willing to back it up by following through on the disciplinary actions expressed and agreed upon within the employee handbook, a dress code means very little. A thoughtful, detailed dress code (and protocol for when it's disregarded) may well save your organization from an H.R. issue that would lead to a loss of money, time, and peace of mind. And when your staff members dress professionally, they just might feel a little more pride in their job and take on a deeper understanding of the influence they have in the patient experience, and they will surely instill more confidence in patients regarding their care while bolstering the image of your practice.

What about the doctor? Does it matter what the doctor wears? A New Zealand study showed that patients preferred physicians to be dressed in semiformal or business casual attire (for men, khakis or dress pants, shirt, tie optional, no coat; for women, a dress or pantsuit, business attire that's comfortable and not too dressy) and a smile. Their second choice was semiformal without a smile, and then a white coat, followed by a formal suit, and finally jeans and casual dress. They were less comfortable with facial piercings and earrings on men. Additionally, though they want to be introduced to the doctor by the doctor's full name and title, they want to see a name badge.[2]

Perhaps you're wondering, just how do I word the part about tattoos and piercings? You want to stay objective and be specific in all areas. In other words, when things are left to interpretation, you are asking for trouble. Below is an excerpt of the dress code for employees of the University of Wisconsin, Department of Medicine describing its policy on tattoos and body piercings:

- Other than pierced ears, jewelry worn in pierced body parts (e.g., tongue, nose, gauged ears, lips, eyebrows, etc.) may not be visible or detectable.
- Tattoos with slogans, graphics, sayings, or offensive wording should be covered (e.g., long-sleeve shirt, gloves, etc.). Managers also have the discretion to require that an employee cover any tattoo(s) or combination of tattoos that could be considered offensive.[12]

CASE STUDY

The Extra Mile, or Not

Ms. Suzanne Socialite decided it was time to finally get the eyelift she'd been wanting for years. A friend of Suzanne's who works for a revered plastic surgery practice told her that J.L. Feinstein, MD, was the best eyelid surgeon in town and that even her practice referred difficult cases to him because of his incredible level of skill. This wasn't Suzanne's first time visiting a plastic surgery practice, and she expected a sleek, beautiful interior and "the red carpet treatment." However, Dr. Feinstein shared his practice with physicians of different specialties, and the office appearance was a striking contradiction to the typical cosmetic practice.

To Suzanne's delight, Dr. Feinstein provided a fabulous bedside manner. He made eye contact, took time to answer questions in full, and gave a sense of genuine care and concern as he sat face to face with Suzanne during the consultation. His assistant and surgery coordinator were both personable and helpful, taking whatever time she needed to calculate her costs, find a good date for her surgery, and go over her pre- and postop instructions. She was given a list of items she might want to buy ahead of time, like an herbal pill that could reduce bruising, Tylenol Extra Strength, and an ointment to use during her recovery.

On the day of surgery, Suzanne's husband brought her, but she dismissed him at the reception area when they told her they were running just a few minutes behind, and she'd need to wait. She was soon brought back into an exam room, and Dr. Feinstein's assistant discussed postop instructions with her—such as, "Don't climb stairs until much later when the meds have worn off because we don't want you to fall"—and a hard copy of instructions, including Dr. Feinstein's cell phone number, was given to her to take home afterward. She was then given the medication that would cause her to go into "twilight sleep" for the surgery; and because the previous surgery had gone a bit longer than expected, she was placed in an open waiting area near the back of the suite to wait.

Suzanne began to feel the medication taking effect, with a sense of drunkenness and difficulty focusing. At the same time, she felt the need to use the restroom. She hurried to do this before she would be completely out. She stumbled to the checkout counter to ask where the restroom was and was directed outside the practice to a shared restroom.

Suzanne barely made it back, and that was all she remembered until she was home hours later waking to puffy, sore eyes that wouldn't close all the way and were terribly dry. She remembered Dr. Feinstein's assistant giving her samples of eye drops and had her husband dig them out of her purse. Then she remembered what she'd been told before surgery. "Wait! How did I get upstairs?" The staff had failed to tell her husband to not let her take the stairs directly after surgery, but thank goodness there had been no accident. Hours later, Suzanne felt miserable, the icepacks she had at home were heavy and not flexible enough to mold to the shape of her eye sockets and bring relief, yet ice cubes were too loose, pokey, and difficult to hold in place. A family member went to the store for softer gel icepacks, but she also found that her skin was so sensitive that towels were too rough to use over the icepacks, so they tried different things and finally found a softer cloth to use.

Because her eyes were so swollen and wouldn't close, the dryness was very uncomfortable in spite of using the sample eyedrops given to her by Dr. Feinstein's assistant. About a day later, she tried using a silky sleeping mask to help keep her eyes closed, retain moisture, and rest—it helped a lot. A friend brought over two round icepacks made especially for eyes that her dermatologist had given her; Suzanne was ecstatic that these even existed! When Suzanne had a question over the weekend, she hesitated but eventually called Dr. Feinstein, and he graciously returned her call and answered her questions, remembering exactly who she was.

She trusted Dr. Feinstein; he seemed to really care. But her experience was very mixed and ultimately disappointing. She wondered if he knew all the ways she could have been made more comfortable, the risk she was put at when she left his office to find the building's restroom without staff seeming to notice, after she'd been given mind-altering medication. She wondered what she may have said or looked like in the open waiting area in the back of the office where patients were passing by while she was under the twilight medication. Had she made a fool of herself? And what about how they told her not to attempt to take the stairs at home until the medication had worn off, but didn't tell her husband?

Suzanne remembered the luxurious terrycloth bathrobe she was given at another practice where she'd obtained cosmetic services, and wondered why a complimentary bag of all the things she was going to need wasn't provided for her by Dr. Feinstein, especially considering the high cost of the procedure. Surely he knew from patients how they struggled and the great tips they had found along the way. Dr. Feinstein's specialty was eyelids. He must know about the small round icepacks; he could have provided samples of Tylenol Extra Strength and the ointment to spare her a trip to the pharmacy—and at a nominal cost to the practice. Was he simply not listening or did patients not tell him, she wondered?

Suzanne Socialite was plugged in around town, she knew lots of women she could refer . . . but would she? She'd spent thousands of dollars on an elective procedure and in the end had satisfactory results, but certainly not a stellar experience. It all could have gone so much better with just a few offerings to cater to the needs of patients. Do you think she could find another plastic surgeon's practice willing to meet her every need next time she's ready to part with thousands of dollars? You bet.

GETTING IT RIGHT

"Do I have to cook every day?" the young man asked his mother on the first day after moving out to live on his own. "No, only on the days you want to eat," she replied. Do you *have* to change the staff's dress of a cozy mixed bag of scrubs? Do you *have* to solve the stroller problem for those young moms bringing in their little ones? Do you *have* to start surveying patients and updating your Web site? No, of course not—only if you want to secure your place as a best practice and strengthen your position in the marketplace. Because, if you don't, it could be in two years, it could be in two weeks, but it's likely another practice will eventually move in on your turf, and it is going to be strategic about gaining market share and meeting patients' unmet needs. So, if you're hungry, learn to cook and do it regularly!

The bottom line is that when we give patients what they really want, we are rewarded with success. Success can come in the form of stellar online reviews, loyal and referring patients, a recognizable brand with community support, happier and more compliant patients, and staff members that are rewarded with positive patient feedback and a sense of fulfillment. You can do this. Take a deep breath, and begin at the beginning; get key players on board, start to prioritize, and make a list—you got this!

It is our hope that you are feeling excited and empowered to start implementing fresh ideas, and perhaps some concepts you had already embraced but hadn't yet put into practice, to improve the patient experience in your organization and give a friendly wave as you pass by the competition on your way to being among the best.

THE PAYOFF

When leaders communicate a no-blame attitude, patient feedback can be embraced by staff as a catalyst to an improved patient experience and increased job fulfillment as the practice thrives. The bottom line is that when you give patients what they really want, without compromising your clinical judgment, you will be rewarded with success

References

1. Wysocki AF, Kepner KW, Glasser MW. Customer Complaints and Types of Customers. University of Florida IFAS Extension. 2012; http://Edis.ifas.ufl.edu/hr005. Accessed June 14, 2013.
2. Thiedke CC. What do we really know about patient satisfaction? *Fam Pract Manag.* 2007;14(1):33-36; www.aafp.org/fpm/2007/0100/p33.html. Accessed June 14, 2013.
3. Capko J. *Take Back Time.* Phoenix, MD: Greenbranch Publishing; 2008.
4. Dyche L, Swiderski D. The effect of physician solicitation approaches on ability to identify patient concerns. *J Gen Intern Med.* 2005; 20:267-270.
5. Bachman J. The patient-computer interview: a neglected tool that can aid the clinician. *Mayo Clin Proc.* 2003;78:67-78.
6. Heisler M. Actively engaging patients in treatment decision making and monitoring as a strategy to improve hypertension outcomes in diabetes mellitus. *Circulation.* 2008:117;1355-1357.
7. New Doctor Harder to Find Than New Significant Other for 29 Percent of Americans: Survey. HuffingtonPost.Com. November 19, 2012; www.huffingtonpost.com/2012/11/19/harder-to-find-find-doctor-significant-other_n_2138083.html. Accessed June 5, 2013.
8. Mehrabian A. *Silent Messages.* Belmont, CA: Wadsworth Publishing, 1971.
9. Brody JE. Well-chosen words in the doctor's office. *The New York Times.* June 8, 2009; www.nytimes.com/2009/06/09/health/09brod.html?partner=rss&emc=rss&pagewanted=all&_r=0.

10. Landro L. The talking cure. *Wall Street Journal.* April 9, 2013; http://online.wsj.com/article/SB10001424127887323362880457834622396074296.html.
11. Medical Patients Rights Act. Illinois General Assembly. www.ilga.gov/legislation/ilcs/ilcs3.asp?ActID=1525&ChapterID=35. Accessed August 8, 2013.
12. University of Wisconsin, Department of Medicine, Human Resources, Dress Code and Appearance Policy. www2.medicine.wisc.edu/home/hr/dresscode.

CHAPTER 9

How Facility Design Impacts the Patient Experience

A patient's first impression is gathered from several touch points. How a patient feels the first time he or she enters your facility is a vital component of that impression. Providing a desirable experience in a space that makes sense in the context of the practice image, as well as providing an efficient environment for the functions of the practice and meeting the needs of the patient base, is not just impressive, but crucial to a thriving, profitable business. It's not just about bricks and mortar—or furniture and paint. Your building has important performance responsibilities. Starting with a well-designed layout and following through with aesthetically pleasing and efficient details will streamline practice flow, improve staff efficiency, and give patients a stellar experience so that everybody wins.

T HE REALITY IS that most people spend more waking hours at work than anywhere else. For those that work in the medical field, the majority of that time is spent in a medical facility such as a hospital, clinic, surgical center, urgent care clinic, specialty treatment facility, medical practice, or diagnostic center. Even though so much time is spent in the work environment, how we feel about that space is usually subliminal and not something we consciously think of. Where you work is just a fact of life. Though some may grow frustrated working in an inefficient facility or confined to a space that is too small to "do the job right"—and they might even gripe from time to time—most eventually accept their work space and figure there isn't much they can do about it. The truth is that the importance of this space, and its contribution to a business' success or demise, is consistently underestimated.

THE IMPORTANCE OF YOUR PHYSICAL PLANT

The physical space you work in is an environment of its own, often neglected and misunderstood in its importance and impact on a practice or other healthcare facility. The physical plant can actually be considered a practice tool. Just like diagnostic and procedure equipment, how well it works is vitally important to the overall performance of the people that use it and the business as a whole. In a medical facility, this means physicians, employees, and patients.

FIRST STEPS FIRST

When planning or evaluating a space, think first of the facility's performance requirements before worrying about its ambience and how it looks because an attractive building that is not big enough or that lacks the proper layout will cost you in lost revenue *every single day*. That's right, no matter how attractive your facility or the décor is, it cannot overcome inefficiencies that cause disruption and waste time like a poorly laid out or insufficient space.

We rarely see a practice build a space that is too large. Decision-makers are far more likely to underestimate their space needs, often due to a focus on budget concerns that do not take into account or encourage growth. In these cases, not enough square footage is acquired, and the mistake is costly in the long run. Failing to recognize how important it is to identify your *real* space and function needs on the front end can result in a need to renovate or expand space long before it was intended, costing far more money than having done it right the first time. Additionally, the inefficiencies of an inadequate space drain a practice of resources every day. All of these contribute to an enormous loss in the long run.

It is important to take a diagnostic approach to examining how well existing space functions—what works well and what is hindering performance and patient service. Compromising performance and service are costly mistakes in the use of time and resources, as well as threatening your ability to be more patient-centered.

When considering how to apply your décor budget—which of course has an important influence on the patient experience as well as that of staff —you don't want to skimp, but it is important to focus the majority of this budget on the reception area. This is a space that every patient encounters. Patients expect this space to be as comfortable and well put together as their own home, or more so. The clinical space décor is expected to be bright, clean, and simple.

IT'S A PACKAGE DEAL

Don't overlook the obvious. Selecting a new space is not just a new suite, but often a new building. That means location, amenities, and parking convenience all need to be considered. In addition, what's the area like? Can your patients easily transition to this new location? How is the signage leading to your suite? Are the neighboring businesses a good match for your practice? A pediatric practice next to a Hooters restaurant might not be a good idea. An orthodontist across from a middle school or a sports medicine practice near a fitness club sounds like a wise choice. When selecting new space think about the site itself, not just the space you will occupy.

CASE STUDY

A Painful Mistake

Heidi Springer, MD, and Timothy Guard, MD, outgrew their rheumatology office space several years before they decided to make the big move and the even bigger investment in a new office. Finally, they were ready and spent the better part of a year looking for new space. The entire practice team remembered how quickly they outgrew the existing office, so they carefully thought about how much space they would need once they added another physician and another provider. They also wanted an infusion lounge to provide extra comfort for the patients. The doctors and their practice manager, Sandra Black, looked at many possibilities, and they ended up choosing an office with great visibility from the highway that was near a major intersection, giving them added exposure and making it easy for patients to find.

Once they decided on the office space they wanted, the design phase took another six months. They looked at drawing after drawing of floor plans, paying close attention to every detail. Sandra and the physicians addressed every shortcoming of their existing space and considered all the aspects of their future needs. The nursing supervisor was involved in the design of the clinical space and paid close attention to clinical flow and communication. Everyone was meticulous in analyzing their space needs and traffic flow, and privacy issues and OSHA requirements were evaluated. Once the floor plan was finalized, Sandra worked closely with the designer to make sure the interior was beautiful and the reception room would be both aesthetically pleasing and comfortable.

At long last, they moved in and were ready to see patients. The reception room was stunning, the administrative staff had plenty of room, the manager now had much needed privacy, and there was a conference room that also served as a staff lounge. The clinical area was spacious with a large nurses' station, more treatment rooms, and a first-class infusion treatment lounge. They were prepared to grow. What they weren't prepared for were their very own patients!

The practice consists mostly of adults, with more than 35% of those being senior citizens. The building they chose is three stories high. And though they are technically on the first floor, the first floor is actually a split-level. The new suite is on the upper half of the split-level. Patients are required to walk from the first floor parking lot, through the general lobby to a 10-step staircase or take a mechanical lift (not an elevator) to get to the suite. Not only is this inconvenient for older or handicapped patients, it's confusing as the suite is still considered part of the first floor. Patients taking the lift would push "2" thinking they needed to go up from what is obviously the first floor, but would end up on the floor above the suite because two levels were named "1." No amount of signage or prior instruction to patients arriving at the office for the first time solved the problem. Patients arrive late, and senior citizens are quick to voice their displeasure. Many of them are afraid to take the lift, meaning they must take the stairs—handicapped or not. It is a painful mistake, and one that could have been avoided.

The practice selected an interior designer that had substantial experience with medical offices, but failed to hire a medical design architect. A medical architectural design firm would have certainly discouraged selecting a space that fails to meet the needs of a large portion of the practice's existing patient population. It was a mistake this practice learned to regret and one that unfortunately can't be reversed or repaired.

FUNCTION FOLLOWING FORM

When designing a medical facility, most practices and architects make the mistake of planning the design before they know how they need the space to function. There is more to the design of a medical facility than its physical plant. It is similar to industrial engineering where you must organize all the functions of the plant to work together in order for the plant to function at its highest productivity.

There is a quote by famous architect Louis Sullivan, which states that *"form follows function."* Consider the reverse in regard to medical facilities, *"function follows form"*; meaning a poorly functioning practice can be put in a very well-designed space, and its productivity will increase, and vice versa. Reaching the *highest* level of production requires well-organized and well-managed practice systems but also a well-designed physical space.

MAXIMIZE PROFITABILITY: FEEDING PROVIDERS EFFICIENTLY

The reason renowned medical space planner and architect Larry Brooks named his firm "Practice Flow Solutions" instead of "Patient Flow Solutions" is because there is so much more that goes into the flow of a practice than patients. Patient flow is really the byproduct of all the other flow systems within the practice. This may be hard to grasp for those that work "in the trenches" because in that case it's often all about getting the patient through the system. In facility planning, however, there are many other considerations in addition to patient flow. For instance, if a practice has a well-designed space but schedules appointments at an impossible rate for the providers, the space (and practice) will seem chaotic, crowded, and inefficient.

In this situation, stress mounts at a rapid rate. What is interesting is that if you look *only* at the floor plan and fail to consider the specific function the practice requires of the space, it can look like an ideal plan with smooth patient flow.

To organize the systems and staff correctly, you have to know the projected potential patient volume of each provider. The general concept we use once we have the data on existing workflow is *the funnel*. The idea is to get all you can out of the doctors' potential (small end of funnel—output), and all the systems and staffing upstream must have a little excess capacity (large end—queuing). This allows a steady stream of patients to the doctor. When providers' time and skills are maximized and time is not wasted, practices become more efficient and profitable.

The physical plant can actually be considered a practice tool.

This small bit of excess capacity upstream (having just more than enough hands and staff time available than is ultimately needed) works for the appointment template, staffing, and space. You do not need a large amount, just a small amount more than the doctor needs or can handle. Regarding staffing, we like to see employees with a little time on their hands so they can make sure the doctor has all he or she needs and that the *next* patient is ready. If we go into a clinic and see staff running around busy, then we suspect the providers are, unknowingly, not using *all* their time wisely. This is because the staff is off doing something and not there to assist the doctors, so the doctors do things that should be delegated or lose time because patients are not ready when they are. Utilizing providers for lower level tasks is inefficient and costs a practice, hospital, or other healthcare system in lost revenue and compromised patient service.

This all ties in with knowing how much space you need and properly designing it, because the more efficient the practice is, the higher patient volume the practice will typically achieve. This means the practice will need more space and that space needs to be arranged to handle higher volumes of traffic. When done properly, the result is a thriving practice with a space that contributes to success and encourages growth.

STRAIGHTENING OUT PRIORITIES

The most important consideration in designing a new medical facility is planning how it should function *before* you start drawing. This crucial step is one that will save you headaches and lost revenue because if you don't get it right, you don't get a chance to go back and do it over. We've seen plenty of practices stuck with a poor design once a build out is finished simply because they didn't hire a professional to help them map out the functional requirements of the facility first. If it doesn't work for the physician, staff, and patients, you will pay the price for a very long time. So start off right from the get-go, and get your priorities in order.

Figure 1 is a guide to help you prioritize the functions of a healthcare facility space—the Priority Pyramid:

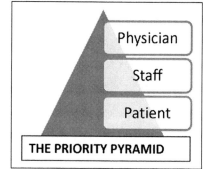

FIGURE 1. The Priority Pyramid.

1. **The Physician.** The doctor is the reason the facility, staff, and patients are there in the first place. Concentrate on eliminating steps and time between patients for providers.

Often we find that managers/administrators start worrying about how long the doctor is in the exam room. It's not their, or our, prerogative to tell a doctor how much time he or she should spend with a patient. The physician knows best. What we have discovered is that any lost time during the patient visit pales in comparison to the physicians' lost time when the space design is not efficient for flow. If the doctors have to walk down a long hallway to a desk or counter space, or if exam rooms are far apart, the clinicians end up taking many steps that would otherwise be unnecessary. These steps equate to considerable lost time and lost revenue at the end of the day.

2. **The Staff.** When staff time is misused, either more staff members are required or staff members are not available when the doctor needs them, and the doctor's time is misused.

3. **The Patient.** We have found that by concentrating on the doctor and staff flow patterns and time utilization, the patient benefits by the practice functioning more smoothly and running on time. Every patient wants to get in soon, get through quickly, and get good care—efficient space planning can help with all three.

Everyone in the practice is important, and the priority pyramid is not a level of importance—after all, without patients there is no need for either staff or physicians. We all need each other. However, if the physicians' needs aren't met, their production isn't optimized, and everyone pays the price. The physicians ultimately provide the care that produces revenue to keep the practice going.

EFFICIENCY: IT'S ABOUT PEOPLE, SPACE, AND SYSTEMS

It is not just about bricks and mortar; an efficiently planned space requires understanding the entire business—the functions, work processes, and flow involved, including:

- Appointment scheduling templates;
- Communication systems;
- Staffing model;
- Individual job descriptions; and, of course,
- The doctors' *potential* rate of seeing patients.

The last item on the above list is seldom given enough value and attention. How fast and how many patients the physician can see over a specific period of time dictates the workflow once the patient is roomed. This is vitally important. We say *potential* rate of seeing patients, which sometimes is far greater than the *actual* number of

149

patients seen. When we discover the potential is greater than the number of patients seen, it's a simple conclusion that the physicians' production is not optimized, thus inhibiting the profitability of the practice and, most likely, patient service.

This doesn't happen because the doctors don't care or are not working hard. It generally means they aren't working smart. They may be taking too many unnecessary steps or being interrupted excessively and unnecessarily. Sometimes they are simply doing tasks that could easily be delegated to support staff. Too often we assume we are working as fast as we can and doing the best we can, when in fact, there may be a way to streamline processes and work to ensure our facility maximizes the opportunity to do so.

The inefficiencies of an inadequate space drain a practice of resources every day.

Part of the problem is that all of us get used to working a certain way in our environment and seldom take a critical look at what we could do differently. When you are thinking about design modification or acquiring new space, one of the best investments you can make is to bring in medical design experts and healthcare management consultants to help guide the process. These experts will provide an objective and critical look at what you can do to streamline flow, improving efficiency, patient service, and profits.

Let's take a look at the impact on a practice that just *one system*, specifically practice communication, can have when poorly organized and managed.

The Communication System

The communication system and habits surrounding communication throughout the organization must be examined when designing space. If the doctor and staff are walking all over the place to deliver instructions and orders, then their productivity will suffer. If a physician is interrupted during clinic sessions, he or she gets behind. If staff members spend precious time looking for someone, then their communication system is weak and time is wasted. The cost of a poorly functioning communication system cannot be easily retrieved, and the practice is likely to experience the following:

- Patients are not going to be happy with delay in care.
- Some staff will probably work overtime.
- The physician and staff will have work that needs attention left at their workstation or desk at the end of the day, so they are already behind when they arrive at work the next day.

This is a recipe for ongoing stress, dysfunction, and loss in profits.

WHY EXISTING WORKFLOW AND SPACE MUST BE EVALUATED

Existing workflow and space need to be evaluated so logjams causing a backup somewhere in the patient flow and the magnitude of those logjams can be identified. This allows solutions to be developed before any new design starts. The evaluation information is also used as a basis for the design.

By determining the magnitude of the logjams and workflow inefficiencies, projections are made that will predict the potential patient volume once solutions are implemented. This is your basic, old-fashioned *time and motion study*. The difference is that the *time study* should focus on the doctors' time first, then that of the staff and lastly the patient. Remember, patients will benefit from good doctor/staff flow, and their experience will be far more satisfying. All too often, practices focus time studies on how the patient or chart moves through the process, when the major problems lie in how the doctors and staff move through the system and how efficiently everyone communicates.

Humans adapt. So the longer a practice is in an existing space, the longer it has had to adapt to the space allocation and layout. What may have started out as a good facility plan for a small practice has turned into a major problem that compromises efficiency and profitability. The space becomes insufficient and inefficient for the practice after years of growth and change. The practice simply keeps functioning without looking at the high price the entire team is paying to stay where it is.

Perhaps closets have been turned into diagnostic spaces, workstations have been converted into exam areas, and so on, even though they are not in ideal locations and compromise work and patient flow. And because the practice slowly grew over time and humans adapt, the physicians do not realize the harm to production that the *new* flow is causing.

By evaluating the existing space and work/communication flow and projecting a potential new patient volume, the space, staff, and equipment needs of the new facility can be projected *before* the design process even begins. Then a more accurate projected cost can be developed. This is when changes can be made and plans can be altered. Then if the budget is not in sync, adjustments can be made or production postponed *before* expensive design work begins.

Remember that the project should be focused on organizing and designing a practice tool that will serve you for years to come—*not* simply making an architectural statement.

CHARACTERISTICS OF GOOD FACILITY DESIGN

One topic that is vitally important when designing an office is patient flow. Practices wonder which design creates a better flow: one-way (linear) flow or a patient flow where patients exit the same way they entered. We are huge proponents of the latter. It is human nature to try to exit a building the same way you enter. When patients exit the same way they enter the office, the space is familiar, they know where they are going, and they are far more at ease. It's sort of like Dorothy in the *Wizard of Oz* and the yellow brick road and feeling in control.

When a practice has one-way flow, staff must constantly show patients the way out of the facility. This creates patient confusion, takes time, and can lead to chaos. When patients exit a different way than they enter, they feel lost and don't really understand where they are in relation to where they started. This forces staff to escort patients out of the office and leaves them feeling a bit insecure.

Making One-Way Flow Easier

There are reasons a practice believes that one-way flow is the best course for its facility, whether it's the nuances of the facility, the size of the practice, or the volume of patients. It has great appeal for cosmetic practices where patients that have just completed a procedure do not want to be seen by other patients coming into the office. Ultimately, the decision for patients to exit a different way than they enter is the owners' to make. If you decide one-way traffic flow is best for your new or renovated facility, there are some steps you can do to make it easier for your patients:

1. Have good signage that makes it easy for patients to understand where they should go.
2. Get staff involved in how patient care and services will be managed without compromising patient flow or efficiency.

PATIENT SERVICES AND SATISFACTION: CRITICAL FACTORS

Most patient satisfaction surveys are conducted based on an encounter date and shortly after the visit. This means patients may

Tips to Improve Function

Here are a few things you might want to consider when designing your space and determining how it will function for your business. These tips could keep you from making a mistake and help you improve patient flow and efficiency.

1. Organize the clinic around exam pods, a group of all the rooms (exam, doctors' workstation, nurses' station, procedure room, etc.) the doctors need while seeing patients. Reducing the physicians' steps and lost time is a profit builder!

2. Base the number of exam rooms on hourly patient volume and exam room turnover time. There is no benefit to having extra rooms full of waiting patients that grow agitated.

3. Evenly distribute the physicians' exam rooms across the hall from each other. This is far more efficient than having three or four on the same side of the hall—it saves steps and improves communication. Align exam rooms with the short end along hall, which means rectangular rooms will be designed to be long as you enter. This brings doorways closer to one another on the hallway. These two ideas reduce the distance the doctors, staff, and patients walk, saving time and increasing productivity.

4. Plan to have every exam room setup exactly the same (unless usage dictates otherwise). This allows the doctors to know exactly where everything is and reduces the chance that they will have to spend time searching for things. This also helps staff stock the rooms quickly because all things will be in the same place in each room.

5. Recognize the importance of hallways. Much like streets of a city, width of hallways in circulation paths must be wider in higher traffic areas where people are coming from the reception room to enter the clinic or are lining up for checkout in an area where people are passing by. It is recommended that in these areas the space be one-and-a-half to two times as wide as the typical hallway, which is typically five feet.

6. Place nonpatient areas further away from the reception area. By placing the staff lounge and other nonpatient spaces further from the reception area, you decrease the need for patients to walk past these areas and bring patient care areas closer, reducing the distance patients and staff have to walk within the practice. This saves time, which increases efficiency and production.

be unable to give an opinion about the physicians' clinical skills or accuracy of diagnosis and treatment plans because they may not know yet the outcome of their treatment. For this reason, surveys most often will cover the following points:

- Whether they were seen on time;
- Attitude of the staff and doctor;
- Discussion of treatment options; and
- Comfort of the office.

In this case, patient satisfaction is more about customer service, not outcomes. This gets back to the heart of the patient-centered practice. There is a payoff for functioning smoothly and efficiently. It contributes to a more satisfying patient experience. When your facility is working for you, the time spent with patients is more focused, allowing clinicians to strengthen the patient-physician relationship. At the same time, the entire practice team is more productive.

IMPROVING THE PATIENT EXPERIENCE

By addressing the functions and needs of the practice, you will improve the patient experience. This provides another advantage: everyone in the practice becomes more efficient when the patient experience is improved. Here are a few ways your space can improve the patient experience:

- Arrange the receptionist duties so he or she can welcome patients face-to-face as they arrive and not be talking on the phone or behind a glass window. This also pays dividends by hastening the check-in process and contributing to improved patient flow.
- Develop an appointment scheduling template that coordinates with the time elements involved for staff and physicians during the patients' visit. This ensures that wait times for patients will be minimized and bottlenecks are less likely to occur.

- Design flow systems and space layout so patients do not back-track or get disoriented during their visit as they walk the path of care.
- Heighten continuity of care and patient service by using scribes/assistants in the exam room, preferably the same staff person that roomed and prepared the patient. This staffer should be able to perceive the physician's needs during the visit. The same staff person will be able to provide any follow-up instructions or ordering of tests once the physician completes the patient visit. This eliminates the need for different staff members to ask the patient the same questions multiple times.

THE WOW FACTOR

We believe strongly that in addition to clearly understanding the importance of design and workflow, the ultimate goal is to create an awesome impression for the patients. We call it the Wow Factor. It's what makes patients feel they're receiving an extraordinary experience. The Wow Factor impresses patients as they find them-selves enjoying their visit from an aesthetic point of view. With the Wow Factor, patients feel they're in a practice that's a cut above the competition, and they automatically assume they are getting more for their money—including quality medical care.

Utilizing providers for lower level tasks is inefficient.

The Wow Factor is our expression for going beyond the typical, tra-ditional experience provided by most practices and clinics. And here is where we want to inspire and empower you with ideas, resources, and a fresh perspective.

To start, you must consider your patients. What are they like? Are they older folks who like to, or wish they could, travel? Are they immigrants who would appreciate a historic nod to their heritage? Are they young executives on the go? Most practices can't put all their patients into one category, but your typical patient base will have some similarities and common needs and interests, and speaking to them through design will definitely wow your patients.

WHAT WOWS *YOUR* PATIENTS?

Though we touched on this in Chapter 8 in the Consider Your Patient Demographics section, it is appropriate to revisit the topic here. Your facility design elements and layout are a big part of meeting the needs of patients and a tool in going the extra mile in showing them your practice is a best practice and convincing them they wouldn't want to go anywhere else.

Walk in Their Shoes

So walk in your patients shoes, metaphorically speaking, and think about their needs and likes. Do those mothers need stroller parking? Do your geriatric patients need extra space for a walker and a smooth floor to push along, free from floor décor like magazine racks and potted plants that may pose a tripping hazard? If your patients are self conscious about the services they receive at your practice, can you give them additional privacy by not making all the chairs face each other in the reception room and having some tall plants between areas? Do spouses or other family members often attend visits? If so, how can you make their wait more meaningful and enjoyable? Would a silent viewing of a National Geographic program or healthy cooking ideas on a flat-screen television be appreciated?

THE THREE COMPONENTS OF THE WOW FACTOR

How might you make your space memorable to patients and visitors? They should expect that healthcare facilities deliver comfort, good

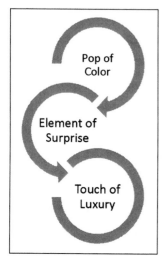

FIGURE 2. The Wow Factor.

lighting, reasonable reading materials, and a pleasant environment, but you can give them an extraordinary experience without breaking the bank. You can provide interest and perhaps intrigue, and make their experience exceptional. It's the Wow Factor (Figure 2), and it consists of three components that aren't difficult to achieve.

We highly recommend hiring an interior design expert with experience in medical facilities. Ideally, someone whose work you have seen and admire. Whoever is selecting the design elements for patient areas needs to be briefed in the desired image of the practice and the patient demographics in order to make appropriate selections and recommendations.

Pop of Color

Providing a "pop of color" means providing a place for the eye to move, creating interest and intrigue that is neither overwhelming or unsettling but just enough to be pleasing. Some ways to achieve the pop of color are through floral arrangements, bright mats on pictures (consider this with black-and-white photos), a small side table in a solid color, or accessories. If the reception room is color coordinated in cool shades of blue and gray, a pop of warm orange would make a statement. If done tastefully, it will not be overwhelming. Of course a youthful, energetic space like that of a pediatric or sports medicine practice may want more color and more "movement" than a practice focusing on elective services for women or a gastroenterologist. What's nice about the pop of color is you can change it and give your space a whole new look without spending the money to totally redecorate.

Element of Surprise

This component of the Wow Factor makes the patient experience you provide truly memorable. Having a few rare ancient artifacts as accessories—perhaps set on a pedestal with museum-like lighting and an explanation of their origins—would certainly make most patients pause in surprise. How about a custom-designed metallic logo and practice name sign on the wall behind your reception staff area or an etched-glass wall feature that exhibits your mission statement? Tickle the ears with symphony music or a fountain. Elegant displays of a collection of shells or antique books or sports memorabilia, or providing a changing and nursing station that is luxuriously and generously outfitted to any mother's needs and wishes could be just the element of surprise to wow your patients. Whatever you do, play to your demographic.

Touch of Luxury

This component of the Wow Factor really cinches the wow. Impressing patients with something they consider a luxury will wow them and speak volumes as to the quality of care they receive at your practice and its value. It's not necessary to overdo this element, just provide it where you can and where it makes sense. Talk with a local florist about having fresh flower arrangements delivered regularly in exchange for their business cards being next to the display, provide water bottles or a custom coffee station where patients can easily brew just one cup of whatever they prefer, a heated coat rack, or the changing and nursing room mentioned above. Any of these would fill this component of the Wow Factor in ways that will set your practice apart from the competition. A warm blanket for patients resting in a dental chair, a tote bag filled with the things your patients will need after their visit, and a luxurious bathrobe with your logo on the front given to cosmetic surgery patients are types of luxuries that speak volumes to patients and can be provided in a way that makes sense when planning your facility design and layout.

YOUR FACILITY, YOUR FUTURE

Your facility is first and foremost a tool of your practice. It must meet certain performance requirements in order for your practice to perform at optimal efficiency and production—period. Beyond function, design and ambiance are important elements of the practice image and patient experience. A word from the wise—in this case Larry Brooks: *"Get it right the first time."* If you are doing a redesign or moving to a new facility, carefully consider all the performance requirements this space must meet while accommodating projected growth. Get an accurate measurement of space needs based on the projected potential patient volume of each provider. And use the experts. Hiring someone whose expertise and loyalty work to your benefit can save thousands of dollars in the long run by retained revenue with optimized efficiency, not to mention avoiding costly moves and remodels that come too soon due to improperly planned spaces.

The authors gratefully acknowledge the contributions to this chapter of Larry Brooks, AIA, President of Practice Flow Solutions and widely known expert in improving the flow patterns of medical practices.

THE PAYOFF

A healthcare facility designed with the goal of maximizing the providers' time and skills will greatly contribute to a more efficient and profitable practice. Practice décor with the "Wow Factor" gives patients an experience that is a cut above the competition, increasing the perceived value of their visit.

CHAPTER 10

Voices from the Field

No one understands the "patient-centered payoff" like those who provide and receive the patient-centered experience day in and day out. In this chapter, you will hear directly from patients and healthcare professionals who have been impacted by this approach of care that reaches far beyond treating a condition with textbook answers and clinical skill. There are also a few glaring examples of when providers fell short of providing this type of care. Be inspired, empowered, and impassioned to give patients what they want most, and reap the rewards that await those who are willing to embrace and achieve patient-centered status.

YOUR PEERS AND THOSE YOU WORK WITH and for have a credibility that can only be earned by living "in the trenches" with you. Patients can tell you exactly what they need and want; what kinds of small differences add up to big decisions for them to stay with a practice, choose a hospital, move on and never look back, or worse—become a voice that turns away potential patients through word of mouth and Internet reviews. Your peers who have found success and fulfillment have the insight and ability to mentor or turn you toward that same success with advice and experience you respect. It is our intent to provide you with voices from the field to do just that—inspire, empower, impassion, and educate you directly from these sources with that unique credibility.

I ONCE WAS LOST, BUT NOW I'M FOUND

Below is a direct, from-the-gut quote from a breast cancer patient just after her first treatment consultation with a board-certified oncologist who was supposed to be the first of several she would interview.

We had been given a list of oncologists to interview and had planned to try to meet at least a few of them. First we would meet with Dr. Ashouri because three people had recommended him. I entered the meeting bracing myself emotionally. I tried to think of good reasons I could avoid chemotherapy. I was guarded because I figured he would talk "over my head," be scientific, and confuse me with facts that don't change anything for me. What happened was quite different.

From his first words with us, to the last, it was exactly what I needed to hear in exactly the way I needed to hear it. His approach was balanced . . . not too many words, nor too few; kindness and compassion with scientific explanations we could understand. He heard my questions and answered them in ways my mind could comprehend and my heart could accept.

I asked him, "Why do we have to make my body really sick for four months? Why can't I just eat healthy, take vitamins, and exercise to make my body stronger?" He answered, "Yes, that is the idea with most other sicknesses, but not cancer. Now that we have seen these kinds of cancer cells already trying to get into your lymph system, it's not a fair game anymore for your normal cells. Chemo will make you feel sick and kill good cells as well as bad cells, but hopefully, when we are done, the battle between good and bad cells will be back to a fair game. You can then start the road to doing all you can to be a healthy person."

He showed me all the years of statistics of breast cancer and treatments and choices. He explained exactly what my cancer cells live on and what drugs will kill my specific cancer. He showed me how even just seven years ago I would have been given a harsher type of drug, but now they know more, and I only need two drugs and not the third harsher drug that was once standard for breast cancer. He explained why he is prescribing six chemo sessions, and not four or eight.

So from the time he entered the room and looked me in the eyes and said, "So tell me your story," even though he had my medical records in his hand, until the end of the visit when my husband and I were crying and he brought us bottled water, he gently and successfully led us into this next step of dealing with cancer.

As we were leaving, our emotions were obvious. My husband and I were both tearful and solemn. The receptionist at the front desk stood up and said, "You look like you need a hug" and came around the desk and hugged us both. We got in the car and agreed we were exactly where we wanted to be, a place where we are viewed as people with needs, not a disease with

163

treatments. It was then that we decided we didn't want to meet any other doctors.

—Beth Bernstein

Notice how the physician's staff member displays the same compassionate approach as the physician, expressing a consistent culture of patient-centered care. As you read Beth's account of this single visit, it becomes apparent why she had received several word-of-mouth recommendations, and likely she will do the same just by sharing with her support network. Perhaps most powerful of all is how her original intent to interview several physicians changed to, "we didn't want to meet any other doctors."

VALIDATION, AT LONG LAST

An elderly woman insisted that something was wrong with her ear. In the days before the Internet, she could not research her condition herself to find answers and was dependent on her family and physicians to find relief. She experienced *years* of frustration and discomfort as one physician after another told her there was nothing wrong with her ear. Even her family began to doubt her. Then she met a doctor who changed everything. Her daughter tells the story below.

Millie, my mom, was an amazing woman, and she lived to be 96. At the young age of 35, she had almost completely lost the hearing in her right ear. With five children still to raise, she was hoping for a miracle. She discovered she was a candidate for a new surgical procedure called fenestration. This was in 1950, and the procedure hasn't been performed in recent decades, so most otolaryngologists don't even know about it. Her hearing was much improved for many years. However, the procedure created special needs for this ear, and with new physicians not understanding the procedure, this posed a problem for mom as she was aging.

You see, the fenestrated ear was prone to fungus and bacterial infections—plaguing her with constant irritation inside this ear. She went to many ear specialists over the years, and each of them told her she must be doing something wrong. She knew better and was frustrated that these doctors discounted her knowledge about her own ear. She would tell them the story about the surgery and that the physician who performed the fenestration explained she would always be prone to infections and that this ear would always need special care. Yet over the years, her doctors told her she was wrong, and after taking a quick look in her ear would say, "Just take these pills I prescribe, and you will be fine." My siblings and I began to doubt her. After all, we thought, the doctor would know best. But the truth is, she wasn't fine; it was a chronic issue, and yet they wouldn't believe her.

When I took her to Sean Palacios, MD, a neuro-otologic surgeon in Las Vegas, she was finally validated. Dr. Palacios is a young physician and one of the few ear specialists in the country that understands the fenestration procedure. Dr. Palacios spoke slowly and clearly. He made good eye contact and offered reassurance and a pat on the hand. He was patient with her, took her claims seriously, and took a deeper look inside her inner ear. He found the source of the infection and cleansed it before putting her on medication for the ear infection. In a follow-up visit a month later, Mom told him her ear never felt so good. He explained that she would need to have the ear cleansed professionally every 6 to 12 months, and if she did so her ear would be far more comfortable and less prone to infection. She never had another infection. Her struggles and constant battle with ear infections was finally over. It's just too bad she couldn't find a physician willing to learn about her condition and give her the care she needed sooner.

—Janice Lyman

Can you imagine this patient's frustration after years of trying to get a physician to understand her condition? Had she truly been heard sooner, had one of her prior physicians looked deeper into her ear, she likely would have found relief much sooner. Imagine the loyalty she had to Dr. Palacios afterward. Surely she told everyone how he'd been the first one able to help her after so many years of being told there was nothing wrong with her ear but an unavoidable infection.

The family of this patient went on to tell us that Dr. Palacios' bedside manner was superb and that his office staff members were personable, professional, and efficient. Dr. Palacios granted us an interview, and here is what he had to say about the importance and impact of patient-centered care.

> *Building a good rapport with patients is the most important aspect of the doctor/patient relationship and in running a successful medical practice. Our entire purpose as physicians is the care of our patients. If a physician doesn't take the time to explain the patient's illness clearly and with empathy, care provided for the patient will be severely impeded. Unfortunately, the course of medical care and reimbursements has shifted, requiring physicians to see more and more patients in a shorter amount of time. If physicians are not careful, their quality of care is compromised in order to meet the needs of the business aspect of their office. The patients suffer initially; and in the long run, the physicians' reputation and practice suffer.*

> *I believe that patient rapport comes down to individual physician effort and whether or not it is a priority to them personally. It is critical for us to connect on a deeper level with patients because our treatment plans are based on information provided by our patients. How open our patients feel they can be with us will determine if they tell us everything we need to know in order to make the proper diagnosis and treatment*

plan. If our patients do not feel comfortable with us, they are unlikely to tell us everything and may not take our advice and recommendations—naturally, this impacts their care and outcomes. This, in turn, reflects on our practice and us.

I have found that establishing a good relationship with my patients and giving them the time they need has not only enabled me to treat my patients to the fullest, but has also built a fantastic referral source and a thriving practice.

The patient-centered movement is a fantastic idea that will benefit healthcare. I believe most physicians will join the movement. The difficult part is balancing the financial aspect of medicine and our time in this ever-changing healthcare system. I do believe things are not going to get easier, but harder with impending changes in healthcare, and that responsibility will fall not only on the physicians but also on the third-party payers.

—Sean Palacios, MD, Board-Certified Neuro-otologic Surgeon

SWEET ROSES AMONG THORNS

A couple whose son is slowly slipping away from them because of an untreatable recurrence of brain cancer is living in their child's hospital room at a nationally acclaimed children's hospital. There are neither words of solace nor thorns of indifference that could possibly be felt through the sadness they endure as they struggle to hold on to every last day and grapple with what lies ahead . . . or is there? In this case, there *were* encounters with hospital staff that impacted them both positively and negatively. Perhaps this tender testimony as told by the child's father will help you to realize the power of the words and attitudes of healthcare professionals in such delicate times.

We sat with our son day and night, taking turns sleeping so that he would never be left unattended. We didn't want to miss a single request, a look of discomfort, a word, a gentle smile, or even one single sweet breath. One day, a hospital staff member in a business suit entered the room. She spoke softly, which we appreciated; however, anyone entering the room was viewed as an intruder unless they were there for our son's benefit. She brought a rolling cart with plastic drawers and explained what was in each one. The top drawers were filled with items for us to use and keep, the bottom drawer had items for us to use but not take. Inside we found a set of Toy Story printed sheets to make his bed look less like a hospital and more like his room at home. There was an electric teapot and variety of teas, cocoa, and coffee; a CD player/radio; a night light for the countertop; a journal; a frame; snacks; laundry soap and dryer sheets; and toiletries.

Clearly they understood what we already knew: we weren't going anywhere. But they also knew that we couldn't possibly be more needy in all our lives. Thinking just beyond the next hour was difficult, our emotions were raw and our minds a blur as we had little sleep and focused so intently on the facts of our child's status and care: what did the doctor last say, when was the nurse last here.

A whirlwind of services, offerings, gifts, cards, friends, family, and hospital staff came and went, but there we stayed. There we would stay to see our boy through, and nothing else mattered. And yet the words, looks, and actions that did penetrate the fog were actually very helpful. Even children's printed sheets that made us smile briefly as we thought of how he'd like that, how much more he looked like himself with that backdrop. Obviously someone knew what kinds of things we'd need—like a tabletop night light as we fumbled in the dark to trade posts in the middle of the night without wanting to disturb our sweet boy, and laundry services we had not been privy to before that time.

Our time in the hospital brought us in contact with many nurses as the shifts would change, and we were there for several weeks. We appreciated the nurses who didn't try to make small talk with us. Perhaps they were trying to be friendly but chitchat felt irreverent to us in light of the extreme turmoil we were in. However, gentle conversations would sometimes arise as the best nurses took their time to care for our son with such respect. They often gave us tidbits of their personal lives as we showed interest and wanted to know those that were providing important care for our son. A mutual respect grew from these short conversations; and after our son passed, we received many heartfelt cards with personalized sentiments scrolled inside.

One nurse remembered our son from seven years earlier, during his first bout with cancer. Though she was not working on our son's floor this time, she brought us a photo taken all those years ago of him and her and another nurse. We mused on how vibrant our son was, so full of life with his bright eyes, full cheeks, and jack-o-lantern smile from losing his front teeth that year. We told her how he'd enjoyed the past seven, healthy years. We slipped the photo into the frame the hospital had provided and displayed it during our stay.

Our last weeks with our son were made more meaningful because of these expressions. To know our relationship with our son and his kind ways had touched the lives of these staff and volunteers meant so much to us. More roses among our thorns.

Unfortunately, there was a time when we were hurt by a flippant remark made by a staff member. Our son was no longer taking food from the cafeteria, yet communications had not *been successful, and we were still receiving daily calls asking for his order. He was now strictly on an IV. You can imagine how difficult it was for us to acknowledge to ourselves that our son was no longer eating. I asked a nurse to notify the cafeteria staff again . . . to tell them that he was now on an IV and to please stop calling us. And she said, "Yeah, okay, we wouldn't want them to think you're starving him!" That remark was neither funny nor necessary. In fact it stung bitterly for this Dad who was wrestling with every decision about his son's care—wanting to do right by him at every turn.*

—Ethan Devine

On a tender and painful journey, words and actions impacted this couple and their ability to cope—as well as their trust in the physicians and staff that surrounded their son's care—in ways that are difficult to even put into words. You may be wondering how a healthcare professional who works with such sensitive cases day in and day out could make such a mistake. But that is the point: simply forgetting the importance of viewing care from a patient's perspective can be detrimental. The result can be hostility, noncompliance, more work for healthcare workers, and reduced quality of care. What is routine to you is not necessarily routine to patients. Yes, it's going to happen that occasionally patients or family members will have their feelings hurt, especially in such an intense setting, but this does not discount how very important it is that staff respectfully consider—and be held accountable for—their choice of words.

RESPECT: MED SCHOOL NOT REQUIRED

Regardless of education level, every patient should be able to expect a basic level of respect for their thoughts and opinions about their own health, right? Here a young, first-time breastfeeding mom relays how an unexpected comment can change an entire experience and leave a lasting impression.

I had just had my first child, a baby girl, and was so excited to be breastfeeding and living near my family during this important stage of my life as a new mom! My baby was just about a month old, and I had a sore breast, with a hot, red spot on it. My mom recognized it immediately to likely be a breast infection that would need antibiotics.

Unfortunately, it was the weekend, so when I called my OB/ GYN, I got the "exchange" and was told I'd get a call back from the "on-call doctor." I was grateful the call came within an hour, but I wasn't prepared for the attitude on the other end of the phone. I explained my situation and symptoms; I told the on-call physician that my mom said it looked like a breast infection. He immediately snapped back sarcastically, "And what medical school did she attend?" I was stunned. I stuttered as I explained that she'd had breast infections and knew what they looked and felt like. He cut me off and asked me what pharmacy I would want to pick up the antibiotics from and then curtly got off the phone with me.

When we hung up, I was dumbfounded as I explained to my husband and mother how the conversation went. As I processed this physician's arrogance, I became angry. Why would he feel the need to belittle my mother and me for simply trying to explain what he could not see over the phone? I didn't tell him I had a breast infection; I suggested that it could be. No, my mother had not been through medical school, but she did nurse three infants, and I am quite sure he hadn't. But that really wasn't the point; he made me feel small, inadequate, and insignificant. As a new mom, feeling exhausted and insecure, that was the last thing I needed. I am an involved member of my community, and you can bet I took my opportunities to share this experience when newly pregnant women asked about different OB/GYNs they were considering for their care. I also let my doctor know about the incident.

—*Jill Chamberlin*

We're not always on our best behavior, but making a habit of respectful speech is so important when engaging with patients. Had this on-call physician kept his thoughts to himself, he could have provided a quick and helpful experience for Jill. Instead, he took a hit to his reputation in the community and with the physician in his call group. Keeping in mind where patients are coming from, both literally (referrals) and figuratively (a place of vulnerability), will serve you well.

WORLD-CLASS NOT ENOUGH

A patient's health journey is sometimes fraught with fear and uncertainty. And even those who have been in "the system" receiving treatments, shuffled from place to place, and given test after test for years seek comfort and relationships to help them cope. Such is the case with this 50- year-old woman who had been accepted into a world-class treatment center that promised her hope of reaching her dream of living long enough to raise her three daughters.

> *"I have not given up on [large, famous cancer treatment center], but I am just considering it. It really is an amazing place, one of loveliness and miracles. But I want to be in a place where I feel known, and I don't really recall the doctor even using my name more than once. He is brilliant, smiley, and detached!"*

—*Karen Humbles*

It is amazing that in the fight of her life, this patient is considering leaving a world-class facility with revered physicians to return to her local specialist simply because she felt "known" there. This testimonial speaks to the incredible power of the physician-patient relationship.

CAN YOU HEAR ME NOW?

A young girl is diagnosed with type 1 diabetes. If that's not hard enough, she struggles to find a way to manage her disease in a way that best fits her lifestyle and reduces the incredible impact it has on her and her family. When she finds what she and her family believe to be the solution, they are met with a reaction from her doctor that throws them a curve.

I was just 11 years old when diagnosed with type 1 diabetes. I didn't even know what that was; I thought it meant I was going to die. Fortunately, someone I knew and felt comfortable with, my pediatrician, gave me this news, and he immediately assured me that I was not going to die. He arranged an appointment for me at children's hospital downtown the very next morning. There I was assigned an endocrinologist, Dr. Colleen Davis. She was older, had a deep voice, a stern nature, and played with a rubber band as she spoke to my mom and me. It was a traumatic day for me already, but her lack of warmth made me feel even more intimidated. We continued with Dr. Davis over some time, hoping her stern, strict nature would help us stay on track as we learned how to manage my diabetes.

Eventually, I grew tired of taking seven shots a day. My mom had to travel to my school and test my blood sugar at lunchtime. I had to answer questions from kids at school, and both my mom and I were constantly preoccupied with my diabetes. I would have done anything for a sense of normalcy. After doing some research, my mom and I believed an insulin pump would give me the normalcy I craved. I found out that my favorite singer, Nick Jonas, used a tubeless insulin pump called the OmniPod. I really liked the idea of using a pump that didn't have tubes hanging off of my body. I was now in middle school, and the last thing I wanted was a long tube hanging off of me when I dressed out in PE.

My mom and I talked to Dr. Davis about the tubeless pump we'd learned about. Immediately she shot us down, "You're too petite," she told me. "It works best on big, overweight men who have lots of fat and skin to cover the pump." Then she went on to tell us all the wonderful things about the pump that her hospital was accustomed to recommending. I felt discouraged and discounted, but in an effort to be open-minded, and of course trusting our physician, we went home and did more research. We read about the features of the OmniPod and saw many positive patient testimonials. We couldn't understand why Dr. Davis refused to consider this pump for me.

Three months later at my next visit with Dr. Davis, we brought up the tubeless pump again. When she started talking about the features of normal insulin pumps with tubing, my mom and I explained the facts that the OmniPod had all of those qualities, but even more. We were sure it was the best solution for me and my lifestyle.

It took us over a year to convince Dr. Davis that the OmniPod was the pump for me. She was stubborn and old-school, wanting only to work with devices she knew. My mom continued to advocate for me, and Dr. Davis finally agreed to let me wear a demo of the tubeless pump for three days to make sure it was something I could get used to. I wore it for four days and loved every moment of it. By this time, there was nothing more that she could do but let me get the OmniPod. This meant my mom coordinating with the device company and eventually the *hospital staff being trained to use and teach others how to use this tubeless pump.*

After I finally got the tubeless pump, we decided it was time to request a new endocrinologist. The hospital assigned me Dr. Mimi Sanders. We found her to be kind, understanding, and forgiving when we made mistakes with managing my pump and diabetes. Before we had felt condemned when we'd make mistakes. At this time, I was playing field hockey as an extracurricular sport. Dr. Sanders shared that she used to play field hockey, so she could really understand and help me with managing my diabetes while I played. She also used to work on the east coast, where OmniPod was first being manufactured, so she was one of the first to learn about the pump and how to use it.

I wish I'd found Dr. Sanders sooner. I was so grateful to have finally found the right doctor, who not only listened to me, but also cared for me.

Without my mom's support, I don't know if I ever would have gotten this pump that changed my life. Dr. Davis discounted my requests and the research we presented to her. Dr. Davis was more interested in doing what she was accustomed to than listening to our needs. This whole experience has enabled me to be strong and to become an advocate for other kids at the children's hospital to have this option. And seven years later, I'm still happily using my OmniPod.

—*Tara Schmidt*

I find it incredible that this young woman, now 18 years old, remembers that in her first visit with her endocrinologist, the physician was playing with a rubber band. At just 11 years old, she picked up on the triteness of this act when she and her mom were scared, intimidated, and overwhelmed with a diagnosis they still knew little about. Tara told us that she and her mother knew that Dr. Davis cared about her, but the doctor's inability to connect and unwillingness to consider solutions other than what she was accustomed to greatly impacted Tara's experience and prolonged her wait for what ultimately brought her freedom, comfort, and convenience.

It's fantastic that this patient went on to advocate for other kids with diabetes, but what if she and her mom didn't have the persistence or the ability to research as they did? Would Tara be going off to college now with unnecessary tubes hanging off her body? How many embarrassing moments at school—questions and looks from peers—would she have had to endure? Had Dr. Davis initially embraced her patient's research and considered the tubeless pump sooner, she'd be the heroine of this story having championed the patient's right to the latest technology when it makes sound medical sense. Instead, her patient eventually moved on to a find a physician she felt would support her better.

NO SMALL THING

We all have an off day from time to time. This patient was having an off *year*, and her experience with a fellow was so impactful that she felt compelled to write a letter to her physician *six months later*, asking her to deliver it to the fellow on her behalf. We thank Linnea Chap, MD, and the patient for giving us permission to share it with you.

> *Dear Doctor,*
>
> *You won't remember me—just one more tiresome old woman with breast cancer whom you had to interview while working with Dr. Chap, asking all those tedious questions about pain, vomiting, etc. You certainly were bored and took no trouble to hide it. It's not pleasant to be treated like that, but I can live with it.*

What I can't live with, and the reason for this letter, is what happened when you'd finished your list of questions. You looked up and asked brightly, "So, how was the surgery?" This was just a couple of weeks after my mastectomy, and I was very sensitive about it. I wonder, if you had just had your penis removed and some stranger asked cheerfully, "How was the surgery?" what your reaction would be. Think about it.

I had really, really wanted to avoid losing my breast. I underwent chemotherapy, which was absolutely terrifying and very traumatic, followed by lumpectomy to try to avoid having the mastectomy. The chemo didn't work, and the lumpectomy could not get the entire tumor, so there were no more choices. Surely nothing can be more horrifying, at any age, than facing the deliberate mutilation of one's own body. Mastectomy is technically minor surgery, but there is nothing minor about its effects, either physical or psychological, on the woman who undergoes it.

Your throwaway question totally trivialized all that I had gone through during the previous six months. I felt as though you had flipped me off. Perhaps this explains why I refused to allow you to examine me.

I need to tell you this because, six months later, it still upsets me that any doctor could be so completely insensitive to a patient's feelings. I suggest that you either take an intensive course in sensitivity training, or move to pathology, where patients' feelings don't matter. Otherwise, you will continue to violate your Hippocratic Oath as you did with me.

Sincerely,

Spring Verity

It is only fair to assume the fellow to whom this letter was addressed had no idea that his apparent lack of interest or empathy was showing through so blatantly. And that is just the point. He was not a nervous, inexperienced resident, but a fellow who had chosen this specialty. What is mundane and tedious to you as a healthcare professional could be one of the worst days of a patient's life, a moment when his or her nerves are on high alert. Did the fellow say something out of line? Did he cross a line of inappropriateness? No. It would be difficult to describe how he fell short without the patient's viewpoint—and yet, it's very powerful. She believed he was bored, detached, and totally out of touch with the patient experience. That's a deadly combination for any practice or healthcare organization.

PERSONAL AND PROFESSIONAL REWARDS

Linnea Chap, MD, a board certified oncologist at Beverly Hills Cancer Center, is maxed out! She sees patients in some of the worst moments of their lives in a bustling oncology practice. In her personal life, she's a busy mother of a "tweener" and *three* teenagers. And yet, Dr. Chap finds time to extend a personal touch in her patient care. Not only does she enjoy it—which is evident by the laughter and hugs she and patients experience during visits—but she reaps the payoffs as well. Hear from Dr. Chap herself, below.

> *As a resident, I was rotating in the oncology clinic with one of my mentors, Steven Rosen at Northwestern Memorial. He mentioned how knowing and remembering something simple and somewhat personal about patients, such as what they do in their free time or a vacation that is coming up, can make them feel special and not like "just another cancer patient." I took this to heart, and it became a part of me. Years later, I told one of the fellows in my clinic at UCLA the same thing. He asked a patient something personal about herself, unrelated to the cancer. When she returned to the clinic three months*

later, and he brought it up to her, her face lit up with delight, which in turn made him feel good as well. A connection was created that went beyond the often-businesslike relationships doctors have with their patients. I've always tried my best to treat my patients how I would want my own family members and friends to be treated. I can't stand the stereotypical description of a doctor with his or her hand on the doorknob during the patient visit.

Although medical schools are working harder to teach bedside manner, it is something that comes more naturally for some. A doctor or physician in training needs to remember how he or she would want to be treated or have a family member treated. This is where I spend most of my waking hours; I can make this a positive experience for me and my patients by building relationships that remain professional but also personally gratifying for both of us. For instance, my patients sometimes refer to me as the "hug doctor." I grew up with a father who was known for his "bear hugs," and I understand the power and warmth of a good hug. It's something I'm comfortable with, and I know how to gauge my patients for when this is a good idea. If I have the sniffles or they do, I say, "OK. Only an air hug today!" I feel a type of friendship with my patients and share in their joys. They even give me advice on parenting since I'm in the trenches with that! Cancer patients, in particular, are terrified; I think that developing a connection with them can soften their journey and also develop their trust. When asked if it's worth it, my answer is YES!

Although losing patients to their cancer battle is gut-wrenching when you've developed a relationship with them over time, the benefits outweigh this hardship by far. First of all, the loyalty and respect I have from patients and my peers keeps my practice thriving. A doctor's income is comfortable but far from what it used to be with all the healthcare cutbacks. With high overhead and poor reimbursement, doctors need to up their volume of patients, which translates to less time spent with them—this is a real challenge. Additionally, many private practices are being bought up by large hospitals, often leaving patients with even more complex issues to deal with in what may feel to them like an abyss. This makes it even more challenging than ever to engage and develop these relationships but it's still possible and crucial to building patient loyalty. I have changed locations twice since being at UCLA. The majority of my patients have followed me each time, insurance allowing. I have a patient who lives in Hong Kong and many who have moved out of state that return to see me for follow-up or continue their active treatment.

I keep a box of notes from patients that I've collected through the years for my children to read some day; it's a personal treasure. Though I haven't found a cure for cancer, my children can see that their mom touched people in a different way, easing their journey with compassion and humor. The personal satisfaction of delivering patient-centered care is an incredible reward in itself. Beyond that, I have gained a very favorable reputation among my patients and peers. I was honored to be named one of the top 1% among oncologists in 2011 by U.S. News and World Report (peer based), and a patient wrote an article about me that was published in the Health Section of the L.A. Times last year. These kinds of things will come to you when you provide authentic patient-centered care. As for my staff, oncology is stressful for all of us. I try my best to praise the staff and try when I can to bring in humor—the best medicine of all!

—Linnea Chap, MD, Board-Certified Oncologist

In our conversations with Dr. Chap, she went on to say that she sympathizes with doctors who are tempted to emotionally "shut off" because it is difficult to feel the ups and downs with patients in such dire circumstances. Beyond that, she explains, she and her peers are being pushed and squeezed to see more patients in less time. She encourages physicians to find a balance that is comfortable and doable for them that also extends the personal touch to patients in a way that makes them *feel* you have all the time they need. This may mean ensuring patient coordinators and office staff are trained to give more personal attention and improving your scheduling template to be more efficient. The rewards have been more than worth it for this passionate physician.

TAKING THE PLUNGE, WITH CONFIDENCE

Patients can be terribly nervous and unsure, even about procedures that will bring them great relief. The ability to put a patient at ease or the mistake to fail to pick up on the fears and uncertainty of a patient can make the difference between scheduling a procedure and another year or two of procrastination. It is a big deal to undergo surgery, accept prescriptions, or take on the expense and time commitment of other therapies. When a patient's concerns are answered with honest, compassionate, and confidently delivered information, you can bet the rate of compliance and scheduling will increase. As in the testimonial below, this works in favor of both the practice and the patient.

I was terrified; I had never been in the hospital before. I had heard horror stories about people that had knee replacements and how they were worse off afterwards. One guy told me he even had to go back into surgery months later. It's funny how you always remember the bad stories, not the successes—I guess the fear kicks in. For five years, I put off having knee surgery. I tried glucosamine, pain pills, and finally a series of injections. Sure, I got a little relief, but eventually the pain would return, and each time it got a little worse. Then last year, I went to Tucson to spend the winter. The pain was so severe that I could hardly walk. A friend told me about a procedure she had that was done by an orthopedic surgeon specializing in knee replacements—it's what he does day in and day out.

I went to see Jay Katz, MD, of Tucson Orthopaedic Institute. I was really taken aback by how he talked to me. I'd been to other orthopedic surgeons over the past five years, but no one made me feel like they understood my pain until now. Dr. Katz was patient and spoke with empathy. He was confident as he told me the kind of results I could expect; that my pain would be gone, and I would have great mobility once I recovered. He told me how long the procedure would take and that I would go home within a day or two. I just knew he was going to help me out. I made my decision that day and never looked back. I wish I'd found him sooner. And believe it or not, I'm actually looking forward to my next knee surgery, knowing the relief it will give me.

Doctors need to know that what they say and how they say it makes a big difference in a patient's ability to feel confident and safe proceeding with treatments or procedures. When they talk with the patient instead of to the patient, we begin to listen and relax.

—Charles Bentz

It's worth noticing how this patient was unwilling to take the plunge of surgery even though he was suffering. Pain is powerful, but fear can be even more powerful. Taking those extra minutes to find out what obstacles the patient has erected in his or her mind and helping the patient scale them one by one is an art that can be learned.

Dr. Katz was able to guide the patient in dealing with the obstacles head-on and boost the patient's confidence to proceed. Everyone wins in this case, and the patient is looking forward to his second knee surgery now.

HURRY UP AND TRUST ME

Barbara Britt, RN, is a nurse care manager caring for children with brain tumors and their families at Children's Hospital Los Angeles. She aims to ease the angst they experience during some of the hardest moments of their lives. Some are struggling to accept a life-threatening diagnosis and rush to sign lengthy waivers for treatment plans. Others have just been told there is nothing more that can be done. And still others are leaving a place they considered their child's last hope without their child. How does a nurse help parents see or hear *anyone* through the fog of emotions on such difficult days? Barbara has more than 40 years of experience and has never stopped learning along the way. We're grateful she took some time to share a small bit of her vast knowledge and experience with us.

> In the work that I do, it's important to quickly develop rapport with patients and their families. It's in the best interest of the patient, the family, and the treatment plan when we have built trust—but we don't have a lot of time to do that. Sometimes parents who have just had a life-threatening diagnosis for their child confirmed are having to sign 30-page "informed consents" that feel as though they are written in a foreign language so their child can begin treatment the next day. This comes following a detailed conference that can take up to two hours, explaining the child's diagnosis and how we propose to treat it. They are still in shock, they don't really feel a sense of choice. They are thinking, "I do this or my child dies." They don't have time to digest all the information or do their own research until they are comfortable with the plan. We've got to

give them more to hang on to than that stack of papers to sign. We can help them by giving them a sense of value, personal investment, and trust. When they sense those things, they can move forward with better coping and hopefully feel that their healthcare team shares their incredible burden. But how do we do this and do it quickly?

One way I do this is to offer something of myself to them. Though a healthcare provider must maintain a level of professionalism and never give a sense that it's "about them" (the staff member), offering a tidbit of personal information extends a sense of mutual trust and value. Anything I share with them about me must be in the interest of enhancing the ability to build rapport and aids in that rapport as we keep the family and their needs in the spotlight. When done in the right moment and sensitively, it says to the family, "I'm willing to take the risk of sharing a bit of myself. I know you are having to share things with me that are private, and I want you to know I'm trustworthy and extending myself back to you in this small way."

When working with the kids, often pets will become a topic of conversation, and I can share with them that I have a Scottie dog at home named Max. We will talk about their pet and its personality and Max's stubbornness. I am establishing credibility and helping the children relate, to improve their experience during care. It's a way to break the ice and say, "We both have a pet at home." We may even relate the pets to the situation at hand. Sometimes it's something more personal, but sharing with patients must be done thoughtfully, with purpose and to give them the best support possible. Some nurses can show that trustworthiness by simply doing exactly what they say they will do. Say you will be back in 20 minutes, and then do it, exactly. Reliably doing what you said you'd do, no matter how small, is a great tool for building trust and confidence.

One of the first things I do with a new family is explain to them our roles. I tell them, "My role is to tell you what you need to know medically in order for you to take care of your child in the context of this new diagnosis." Then I explain to them, "You are our best expert on your child that we have on our team, and I need you to tell me how we can fine-tune our plan so it works best for your family." You see, when a parent is told their child was walking around with a brain tumor for months and they didn't know, they sometimes have an internal dialogue that goes something like this: "How could I have missed it? I did I not know, I'm his/her parent! What kind of mother/father am I?" It's a real confidence-sucker, and I want to build that confidence back up empowering them to contribute to the benefit of the patient, family, staff, and treatment plan. I remind them that they are the experts on their child, and we are a team, partnering together.

We call it family-centered care. In order to facilitate these roles we, as healthcare professionals, cannot assume that we know what's best for families. We need to involve them and ask them. In some hospitals or with some professionals, there is sometimes an underlying sentiment that says, "They can't adhere to the rules of engagement because they are out of control right now." Even though they are in a state of despair, their input is vital to meeting their needs. And when we make it difficult for them to reach us or to communicate with those they trust, they will become more panicked.

It's important to play to the majority—most families want to respect our roles and our time—not the minority, the one in a thousand that will abuse the access we give them. I give families my cell phone number with an explanation of the days and hours that I work and am available to them and that I am not their first call if there is a medical problem (there is always a doctor on call for that). There are so many new people that a family will meet and a learning curve of how the hospital works. It's such a difficult time, just giving them my phone number gives them a tether to someone on the inside of the hospital who also understands just how much their world has been up-ended. There are some issues that to a parent are urgently important. It may not be a medical emergency, but for them to have their concern or question answered swiftly, by someone who knows their child and their situation, can save them a night of fretting That's what I can do for them, as their nurse care manager. That's what that phone call is for.

Once a young boy passed away in our hospital; his mother had mostly cared for him. The female members of the family were primary caregivers in their culture, in particular his mother. Though we have chaplains of every faith available for our families, we were told of a requirement we'd not dealt with before. The family was of a faith that required the father, who had largely been distanced from the child's care until now, to prepare the body of his son for burial with pure white linens. Not only this, but it had to be done within hours. Do you know how hard it is to find white sheets with no logos or stamps on them in a hospital? I tried my best and then realized they would need to be purchased outside the hospital.

I called one of our volunteer families. These are parents who have had a child in our care in the past and who have formed a group and are ready to do anything we need at a moment's notice, even though they will not know the patient or the situation. They understand what these families go through. The husband immediately went to Target to buy the white sheets I needed and swiftly drove to the back of the hospital where I met him to grab the sheets and deliver them to the family as quickly as I could. The father of this child was stepping up to do his duty and fulfill his role in the family by performing this last duty of care for his son. Did I have to do this? Would I ever hear a word of complaint if I let them handle it on their own? No, of course not. There are no sections in any employee handbooks about this.

It is simply a part of the culture of the nurses and hospital I work for. Parents are going to mourn their entire lives; we want to ease the grieving process for families. We deeply respect their values and beliefs whether or not we share them. I did not want one of those family members to have to go to the store that day, in a fog of emotion. That is not what I wanted to be a part of their memory. It brought me great personal satisfaction to deliver this compassionate care that goes beyond any clinical skills taught in nursing school.

You ask me what the payoff is. It's deeply personal for me and most of the staff that I know. It's a principle we hold to, but beside the personal sense of satisfaction and the gratitude we often get from families, there is a payoff for the organization as well. We have families that go out and tell others, "If you want your child taken care of, you go here. Not only will you have the best medical care, you will have an incredible experience with the staff." Our hospital honored the cultural and religious values of that boy's family by giving me the freedom and resources to assist them when I could.

—Barbara Britt, RN, MSN, Nurse Care Manager,
   Children's Hospital Los Angeles

Day in and day out, nurses like Barbara, physicians, and other health-care staff are providing patient- and family-centered care that goes far beyond meeting the clinical, medical needs of patients. These are the people who impact patients' lives, affecting the climate of healthcare delivery. Whether it's simply a sense of being known and heard, or something as important as having one's religious traditions honored during a traumatic life event, these seemingly small gestures and attitudes have enormous impact on the landscape of healthcare by giving patients something to rave about; a place to call their medical home; and somewhere to refer their friends and loved ones, which in turn boosts the reputation of the organization from which the care was received, the providers and other staff, and healthcare in our country overall.

"There is no profit in curing the body, if in the process we destroy the soul."

—*Samuel Golter, Former Executive Director, City of Hope*

THE PAYOFF

Your peers have earned credibility by living "in the trenches" with you, and patients can provide insight into what kinds of small differences add up to big decisions for them—like when to stay with a practice or hospital or move on and never look back. Their insight can influence your success with advice and experience you respect. Reading their personal stories should leave no doubt in your mind that a patient-centered approach will help you pave your own path to success and fulfillment.

CHAPTER 11

Twenty-One Things You Can Do *Now* (Without Breaking the Bank)

It's an old cliché that "it's not about the destination, but the journey," and it's true when talking about the patient-centered payoff too. Becoming a patient-centered practice, hospital, or other healthcare system is an ongoing process requiring flexibility as you continue to change and improve to meet the needs of patients. This chapter is designed for those who need help in narrowing their focus and getting started. Perhaps your facility is patient-centered already and is ready to take it "to the next level." You can use this checklist as a rating system to give yourself a progress report. Remember, if you are moving in the right direction, your patients, staff, and referral sources will notice the change; and as it continues in earnest, the payoff will become evident.

If you're feeling excited but overwhelmed with ideas of how you want to implement the information in this book, this chapter is for you. It's a simple list of recommendations that you can begin to implement immediately without an enormous amount of time or money—but that have a big impact! You will need to prioritize, you will need to stay motivated, and you will need to get your team on board. That may well mean having staff members read this book or portions of it now so that they will "know where you are coming from." The lists below are grouped by categories: practice image, office culture, and patient experience. It's important that you prioritize which items you want to focus on—those that make the most sense based on need or ability to quickly implement.

PRACTICE IMAGE

1. Clean house.
2. Improve staff attire and require name badges.
3. Improve phone access.
4. Review your practice logo and brochure.
5. Say good-bye to the sign-in sheet.
6. Claim your online space.
7. Perform a facility facelift.

1. **Clean house.** Cleaning house refers to literally cleaning up your space, the clinical and the nonclinical. That means a deep cleaning of flooring, baseboards, and window treatments, and making repairs to bathroom stalls that no longer stay locked or to that chipped tile in the reception room. You may have grown accustomed to seeing some of the wear and tear, but patients notice dingy or unkempt areas and equate them with a lower standard of care. Chapters 8 and 9 provide more details on improving the office appearance.

2. **Improve staff attire and require name badges.** Although there is an initial investment, buying practice uniforms, matching scrubs in practice colors, or a polo shirt with an embroidered practice logo is a fast and forceful way to upgrade your practice image. Not only will patients sense an organized, professional healthcare team image, but your staff will *feel* more professional and attain a sense of pride and belonging. Remember, a name badge is a must: a big, easy-to-read font should spell out employees' names with credentials. Including the practice logo on the badge is a fantastic way to continue to brand the practice. For specifics on dress codes and name badges, see Chapter 8.

3. **Improve phone access.** From large corporations to mom-and-pop shops, you find businesses accessible by phone during business hours. So why is it that patients sometimes can't reach their physician's practice during the lunch hour? It makes good business sense to keep your phone lines open during business hours. Patients feel frustrated when they need to get through and can't. Sometimes they have only their lunch hour to get this important task done, and they may be worried about a test result or a sick child. Read in Chapter 5 about how we helped a practice make this important change to better meet patient needs.

4. **Review your practice logo and brochure.** If you have them, review them. Are they outdated? Are they communicating the image and information you need to convey and that patients are attracted to? Does the practice brochure communicate your values, highlight the providers, and give pertinent information that's easy to read? If you don't have them, it's time to talk to a graphic designer. See Chapter 3 for more on branding.

5. **Say good-bye to the sign-in sheet.** The sign-in sheet is one of our personal pet peeves. Patients come at an appointed time and are on your schedule, so they deserve to feel like you are expecting

them. Greeting them personally does this. A sign-in sheet gives your front desk permission to ignore your patients upon entering. The bottom line is: it sends the wrong message. You can do better. This was also discussed in Chapter 8.

6. **Claim your online space.** You can begin by doing an online search of your practice, providers, or facility, as well as using general terms like "pediatrician in Oakville, California" to find sites you are not coming up on. What sites need updates, photos added, etc.? Refer to Chapter 4 for more in-depth information on claiming your online space. Take control of your online reputation! It's only costly if you *don't* do it!

7. **Perform a facility facelift.** A facility facelift is similar to cleaning house, but this is when you decide it's time for a fresh look. Are the drapes circa 1989? How about that artwork in the reception room—would you be excited to hang it in your living room? Do your reception area chairs look up-to-date and meet the physical needs of patients? A budget-conscious redo is possible with the assistance of an interior decorator or redesigner who specializes in using what you have first, then building on it. New flooring, fresh paint, and window treatments go a long way, but it's important to have a long-term plan so that no money is wasted when choosing fabrics, colors, etc. For more ideas about making facility changes that patients will appreciate, see "Consider Your Patient Demographics" in Chapter 8 and "The Three Components of the Wow Factor" in Chapter 9.

OFFICE CULTURE

1. Develop or review your mission statement.
2. Hold a team discussion.
3. Survey patients.
4. Use a mystery patient service.
5. Conduct a customer service workshop.

   6. Set goals for improving patient survey scores.

   7. Survey employees.

1. **Develop or review your mission statement.** Developing your practice mission is an important step in defining your identity as a practice, building your brand, and then meeting your optimum potential. By defining a specific mission that is deliverable through the daily actions of staff, you create a means to measure and improve upon that delivery. Read more about crafting your mission statement in Chapter 3.

2. **Hold a team discussion.** Once you have honed your mission statement, it's crucial that you get your team on board. A brainstorming session to identify specific ways staff members *do, can,* and *will* deliver on the mission statement will enhance the buy-in and team culture among the staff. It's essential to the team atmosphere to encourage and incorporate staff input. Be sure at some point to communicate what is expected and integrate it into future benchmarks and reviews.

3. **Survey patients.** Surveying patients is not as difficult as it may sound. If you have patients' e-mail addresses and permission to use them, enlist the services of an online e-mail survey provider. Another way to gain this valuable feedback is through a short postcard-sized survey (we recommend about four questions and space for comments) that patients fill out after their visit and place in a box so that the surveys remain anonymous. Read more about surveying patients in Chapter 8.

4. **Use a mystery patient service.** A mystery patient service will provide professional feedback that goes beyond what you and your patients will pick up on or be able to articulate. A mystery patient service will include recommendations that you may not have considered and may validate your suspicions—including

that you're doing a great job in many areas! Chapter 8 discusses the mystery patient service in detail.

5. **Conduct a customer service workshop.** Providing your staff members with a customer service workshop enables them to brush-up on skills and revives their motivation with new ideas and reminders of how to deliver top-notch patient-centered service. Perhaps you have a specific concern, and you need a consultant to work through that with the staff or find creative solutions to improve service. If an expert workshop isn't an option, you can have your staff read one chapter of this book a month. In a monthly staff meeting, members can share three ideas they'd like to see implemented from the chapter that would bring your practice patient-centered payoffs. Chapter 1 talks about the importance of investing in training staff on customer service.

6. **Set goals for improving patient survey scores.** "Aim for nothing and you will hit it every time,"[1] a quote by Zig Ziglar, speaks to the importance of setting goals. They can be revised as your practice evolves, but set some goals *now* to keep the team motivated and the customer service delivery measured. A goal might be that you want survey results to improve by a certain percentage when measured again in six months. For example, you may want to strive for a 95% "excellent" or "yes" score for the survey question, "Were you greeted by name when welcomed into our back office?" or "Were you greeted when you reached the reception desk?" Chapter 1 discusses patient satisfaction surveys and measurements in detail.

7. **Survey employees.** It's easy to forget that employees are really the first customers of managers and other practice and organization leaders. When employees' needs are met and they feel valued, they are in a better position to meet the needs and exceed the expectations of patients. Find out what your employees really

want by asking them, but give them the freedom to be honest by providing an anonymous form of surveying. Then respond to their feedback with clear communication and positive changes when possible, which builds trust between staff and leadership.

PATIENT EXPERIENCE

1. Evaluate the creature comforts.
2. Make their visit "me time."
3. Wow them in the welcome.
4. Provide a care package.
5. Implement healthy distractions.
6. Improve communication.
7. Always ask the question, "Is there anything else . . . ?"

1. **Evaluate the creature comforts.** We are referring here to things that make your patients' visits to your practice free from discomfort or frustration. Patients being unable to find your suite because it lacks proper signage is a negative experience you don't want associated with your practice. Can patients easily get out of the waiting room chairs? Are preop instructions given at the check-out desk and overheard by those in the reception area? A patient survey and mystery patient service can help assess where you can improve in this area.

2. **Make their visit "me time."** Going beyond comfort and making the visit feel more like "me time" for patients makes your practice irresistible! Provide your patients with things like a gourmet coffee station, a chilled water bottle, a soft cloth gown, or a warm blanket and ear buds with music during a procedure, and you're likely to seal the deal on patient loyalty and get patients talking about you out in their communities!

3. **Wow them in the welcome.** The greeting patients receive upon entering your practice can set the tone for their entire visit. We've

195

heard patients tell us privately that they like their physician but are considering switching because they feel like the receptionist is a guard dog. Ditch the glass window, and give open-access to patients. Provide eye contact and a warm welcome to each person entering. We recommend that the receptionist not be plagued by phone calls. A designated staff member to triage calls away from the desk is ideal. Visiting patients should take precedence, yet callers shouldn't be stuck on hold.

4. **Provide a care package.** Provide a care package for patients who leave your practice with small needs that you can easily meet. Ease their experience by providing samples and small items that save them a trip to the store. You likely know what they need and can get more ideas from patients themselves in creating a goody bag that truly makes patients feel taken care of. Some practices provide a welcome package (e.g., for expecting mothers at an OB/GYN practice), and others may give a seasonal goody bag. This topic is also discussed in "The Extra Mile, or Not" in Chapter 8.

5. **Implement healthy distractions.** Healthy distractions for patients are easy to implement. If you have a procedure room, provide soothing art and color on the walls. You may even provide soft music to ease nerves. By supplying fresh reading material and something creative for patients and those that accompany them to do, you can reduce perceived wait times while improving the patient experience. More ideas on this can be found in "Consider Your Patient Demographics" in Chapter 8.

6. **Improve communication.** Improving communication may sound vague but can actually be broken down into specific gestures and measurables. For example, using the patient's name upon entering the exam room or finding out a small personal fact to jot down and ask about in a future visit (e.g., an upcoming vacation or a child going off to college) are ways to show patients you care

about them as individuals. Improving communication not only enhances the patient experience, it can improve care, compliance, and outcomes. A breakdown of ways to improve communication can be found in Chapter 8.

7. **Always ask the question, "Is there anything else . . . ?":** Always ask this important question, and you will reduce phone calls to the practice after visits and give patients a sense that it's really all about them. When a clinician asks, "Is there anything else you'd like to discuss?" before leaving the patient, it gives the patient an opportunity to voice concerns and questions about his or her health. This can lead to a more complete picture of the overall patient for the provider, and may lead to the patient seeking care for other issues. When checkout staff ask, "Is there anything else I can do for you?", it gives patients an opportunity to have their questions addressed regarding insurance, payment, and office protocols on subjects like scheduling or records.

POSITION YOURSELF FOR THE PAYOFF

Start now! You'll never be more inclined to put the knowledge, inspiration, and insight that you gained from reading this book into action than you are right now. The longer you wait to implement even just one of these recommendations, the less likely you will do it at all—and your time and monetary investment in this book will not reach its full potential. Find one thing you can start setting into motion, today. When it's completed or you feel ready to take on another, move on down the list. Trying to tackle too much at once may overwhelm you and your staff and could lead to incomplete implementation. We've broken it down here to simplify the process for you. Prioritize and check off a list to get a sense of accomplishment.

If you can hire professional help to implement or assess your needs, make that call today to get the ball rolling. If you cannot make that investment, do what you can now with the budget you have by getting your practice staff on board and moving forward. Your patients and staff will be positively affected as service improves and the culture and environment is enhanced. But the long-term payoff will become evident with time as you see positive improvements such as increased referrals, decreased attrition, and a more satisfied staff giving its best day in and day out.

THE PAYOFF

Put the knowledge, inspiration, and insight that you gained by reading this book to work ASAP by identifying one idea you can start setting into motion today, and continuing to take positive steps to improve the patient experience and your organization's culture and image. The long-term payoffs are increased referrals, decreased attrition, and more satisfied staff members giving their best, day in and day out

Reference

1. Ziglar Z. Ziglar.com. www.ziglar.com/search/aim. Accessed July 22, 2013.

CHAPTER 12

The Patient-Centered Practice Now and in the Future

The patient is at the center of the medical practice's very purpose, and the relationship between the physician and the patient is of utmost importance. If you ask any number of physicians, allied healthcare professionals, support staff, or administrators to define what it means to be patient-centered, you are bound to get a broad array of answers, many of them based on personal opinion. Furthermore, if you ask patients and their families this same question, their answers will be strikingly different from those of the healthcare professionals that treat them. Most healthcare providers do not understand patients' perceptions of their care and what is important to them.

WE NEED TO ATTEMPT to move from *what's the matter* with our patients to *what matters* to our patients, says James Rickert, MD,[1] a board-certified orthopedic surgeon in Bedford, Indiana. What patients want from their physicians is a personal relationship, communication, and empathy. Patient-centered care creates a partnership between the physician and the patient that makes the patient feel valued. It improves communication, clinical outcomes, and patient satisfaction and reduces healthcare costs through increased patient adherence and better disease management.

PATIENT-CENTERED CARE TAKES CENTER STAGE

Patient-centered care has been in the spotlight in discussions of quality for quite some time. In fact, it was identified as one of six specific aims for improvement, as reported in the Institute of Medicine's *Crossing the Quality Chasm* report written more than 10 years ago.[2] The report defines *patient-centered* as providing care that is respectful of and responsive to individual patient preferences, needs, and values, and ensuring that patient values guide all clinical decisions. *Patient-centered* or *patient-centric* is commonly included in the vernacular of healthcare planners, institutes, politicians, hospital executives, and public relations representatives. Many of the discussions about patient-centered care miss an extremely important element—the revolutionary meaning of what is means to be patient-centered. The originators of patient-centered health care were well aware of the moral implication of their work, which was based on deep respect for patients as unique living beings and the obligation to care for them on their terms.[3]

Understanding what it means to be patient-centered is a complex process as it intends to recognize patients in terms of their own

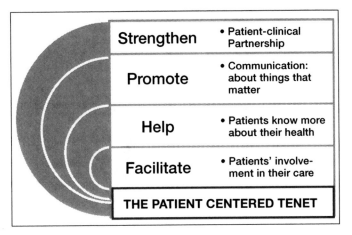

FIGURE 1. Patient-centered tenet.

social worlds. This means throughout the patients' healthcare experience, they should be respected, listened to, informed, and *involved* in their care. The ability to focus on individual needs and apply evidence-based medicine is meant to improve the healthcare of the population. How to accomplish this has been much debated, with proponents of evidence-based medicine now accepting that a good outcome must be defined in terms of what is meaningful and valuable to the individual patient.[1] It is important for healthcare planners, executives, and providers to clearly understand that their efforts and actions are *not* patient-centered unless those actions strengthen the patient-clinical relationship, promote communication about things that matter, help patients know more about their health, and facilitate patients' involvement in their own care (Figure 1). This tenet must be at the forefront of every healthcare organization's intentions with executing a patient-centered program and setting metrics to measure the value and success of these efforts.

GOVERNMENT TAKES A POSITION

The Centers for Medicare & Medicaid Services (CMS) has made the patient experience its business, and accountability is being built into the system. The government has taken the patient experience to a new level by establishing specific standards of expectation. The process began a few years ago with hospitals, but is migrating throughout the healthcare system. Physicians are finding their payments being adjusted based on how well they are reporting care on Medicare patients. In order to receive maximum reimbursement, physicians need to comply. Electronic health records contribute to better reporting, increased compliance, and the ability to receive maximum payment. Other payers are looking at CMS initiatives and are also developing standards that will impact how healthcare providers are paid.

HOSPITALS TRANSFORM

Hospitals are now being scored on their performance and Medicare's Value-Based Purchasing (VBP), which influences payment. Providers must dedicate added attention to the patient experience within the VBP program reflected in hospitals' HCAHPS (Hospital Consumer Assessment of Healthcare Provider and Systems) scores. The scores will determine payment, with 30% of the total performance score based on the patient experience of care dimensions through the year 2015. The remaining 70% of the performance in 2013 is based on the clinical process of the care domain's eight core dimensions. In 2014, the 70% will be split between outcomes and core measures; and in 2015, the 70% weighted value will be based on outcomes, core measures, and efficiency. Hospitals are given points for achievement and improvement for each measure or HCAHPS dimension. These methods of measuring the various aspects of a patient's medical treatment are designed with the intent of improving healthcare of the population and, inevitably, controlling the cost of care.

PATIENT EXPERIENCE OF CARE DOMAIN

There are eight HCAHPS dimensions used to evaluate the patient experience in the hospital setting:

1. Nurse communication;
2. Doctor communication;
3. Hospital staff responsiveness;
4. Pain management;
5. Medicine communication;
6. Hospital cleanliness and quietness;
7. Discharge information; and
8. Overall hospital rating.

Hospitals around the country have made the essential adjustments to address these issues in the past few years, but the providers that influence the hospital's scorecard present challenges. Many physicians in private practice are not accustomed to being monitored for the patient experience in a meaningful way. They certainly understand the need for peer review and recognize that government and private healthcare plans are examining patient satisfaction, but they haven't felt the financial implications in the past. Some of them don't have a clear understanding of the measures that will dictate financial rewards. Now many of them are concerned about how much control government and insurance plans will have over the future of the healthcare delivery system, how they practice medicine, and how they care for their patients. They wonder if the doctor-patient relationship is being compromised in the process, as evidenced in The 2012 Survey of America's Physicians conducted by The Physicians Foundation discussed in Chapter 7.

PHYSICIANS' QUALITY MEASUREMENTS

The Medicare-Medicaid and SCHIP [*State Children's Health Insurance Program*] Extension Act of 2007 authorized CMS to launch the Physician Quality Reporting Initiative (PQRI)—the first nationwide effort by the government to link physician financial incentives to quality reporting. Eligible professionals reported quality measures on a claims basis in order to receive as much as a 1.5% bonus of their total Medicare charges.

CMS established the Physician Quality Reporting System (PQRS) through the Medicare Improvements for Patients and Providers Act of 2008, making the Physician Quality Reporting program permanent. Eligible physicians who elect not to participate or who do not collect and report their data successfully will be penalized in 2015 and 2016 with reductions of 1.5% and 2% respectively.[4]

> *Patient-centered care creates a partnership between the physician and the patient that makes the patient feel valued.*

The 2012 PQRS includes 210 quality measures; 26 of these were new to the PQRS program. Of these 210 measures, 22 are Prevention Quality Indicators. Many of the core measures focus on monitoring patients with chronic conditions and disease management. Such measurements confirm that prevention and early detection are key components to a healthier population and reduction of healthcare costs.

Physicians and medical practices throughout the nation will benefit by understanding PQRS core measures. The participation and adherence to these CMS guidelines will allow physicians to maximize income, while meeting quality standards of care that are intended to improve care quality, decrease complications, and reduce healthcare costs.

LEADERSHIP'S ROLE IN THE PATIENT EXPERIENCE

Hospitals and healthcare leaders face the challenge of addressing the patient experience in a systemic way in order to empower the key players and make a meaningful difference. It begins with messaging; how leaders communicate and demonstrate involvement in improving the patient experience. In the end, how well outcomes are improved will tell the story. Here are a few essential steps leaders can take:

1. **Promote staff understanding.** Set up programs to help staff learn how the patient experience relates to outcomes and finances.

2. **Demonstrate your commitment.** Be visibly involved through communication and actions that continually show intent to improve the patient experience. Be consistent in this effort.

3. **Educate and support staff.** Provide them with the tools and training to succeed and be constant across the organization. Help them understand what you expect, and give them the means to succeed.

4. **Manage the score card.** Communicate what will be measured, and share the scores. Celebrate when achievements are made, and involve staff in developing methods to improve scores where performance is not up to par.

5. **Coach.** Every team needs a coach, and executive leaders understand this, but it is not only the role for those at the top. It must seep into the culture of the entire organization and be an important role to everyone in a supervisorial or training role.

6. **Attain best practices.** Be explicit in what you intend to achieve and how it will be accomplished. Implementing best practices and staying on course is often the most problematic challenge that leaders face, whether in the hospital, academic faculty practice, integrated delivery system, or private practice. It can sometimes be difficult to stay on course when political issues emerge or there is resistance from key stakeholders.

Leaders have the ability to set the stage for success, demonstrate their commitment to being patient-centered, and instill a sense of pride and hope throughout the organization. The entire team depends on the leaders' inspiration and example.

TABLE 1. Shifts in Managed Care

Then	Now	Next
HMOs: Traditionally, patients couldn't go to doctors and hospitals outside their HMO.	Narrow networks: These are often tiered so patients get bigger out-of-pocket charges if they go to providers that aren't in the top category, then even larger bills if they go completely out of the insurer's network.	New plans emerge: Insurers are creating plans built around particular healthcare providers that they employ or partner with.
Prior authorization: Doctors had to get permission from the insurer beforehand for certain treatments, or they wouldn't be covered.	Networks continue: Insurers say the use is targeted narrowly, and they are working with doctors to make it less onerous.	Changed payments: Insurers say payment methods that reward providers for efficiency and quality may decrease the need for policing.
Improved medical outcomes	Improved career satisfaction	Increased productivity

Data from reference 5.

MANAGED CARE'S SHIFT

The managed care revolution of the 1990s has not been forgotten. It forever changed the healthcare delivery system. There were many failures and excessive costs, and it resulted in fewer, but larger healthcare insurance companies. Over the years, managed care has changed significantly, but one thing is certain—managed care isn't going away anytime soon. It's big business; and like most big businesses, it wants to succeed and it wants to control rising healthcare costs. Table 1 demonstrates a few of the most obvious shifts in managed care as presented in a *Wall Street Journal* article.[5] Insurers say current versions of old approaches are driven by better information, which helps them focus on improving care, not just saving money, according to the Journal story. The table reveals that the next initiatives in managed care are designed to create insurance built around healthcare providers they *partner with* and to change doctors' payment methods to reward efficiency and *quality measures*. So Medicare is not the only one that is scrutinizing what hospitals and physicians are doing and closely monitoring outcomes.

The *Wall Street Journal* featured an entire section in its April 16, 2012, edition, entitled "Innovations in Health Care," that included an article on analytics in healthcare.[6] According to the Journal, crunching the numbers can pay off in both better care and lower costs. These numbers drive decisions. WellPoint has partnered with IBM to create a supercomputer. The data-crunching technology will be used to help suggest treatment options to doctors, based on medical records, research databases, and other sources. Memorial Sloan-Kettering Cancer Center in New York is working with IBM to build a tool for cancer treatment that will draw on patient histories, the center's clinical knowledge, and molecular and genomic data. Analytics provides hard data; and the deeper you drill, the more specific information can be gained and with the right intent, be used to advance the practice of medicine and improve population health management.

The Internet and the capacity to use research more effectively changes the face of medicine and how physicians and hospitals will work in the future. Analytics plays a big role in managing healthcare, but analytics doesn't come in contact with the patient—you do. Those of you that actually interact with the patient have an enormous responsibility to and effect on the entire patient experience. Take this seriously, and use it wisely.

PATIENTS AS PARTNERS

The primary purpose of the patient-centric movement is to keep the focus on patients and their needs. Prevention, early detection and intervention, improved patient compliance, and better outcomes rely on being more patient-centered and creating an ideal patient-

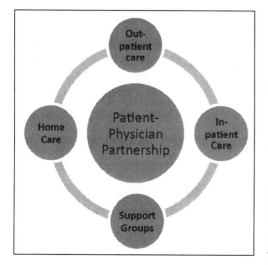

FIGURE 2. Patient-physician partnership.

physician partnership. This partnership expands to other healthcare personnel and providers that work with physicians (Figure 2).

Nurses in the hospital have an amazing influence on how patients feel during their hospital stay. It doesn't take much to rock the patient's boat if a nurse is cranky, but a cheerful nurse will brighten a patient's spirits and goes a long way in creating a positive experience that results in a cooperative patient. The physical therapist that uses good coaching skills will have patients that listen closely, follow directions, and are encouraged to do their exercises consistently, resulting in better outcomes.

Patients are the core of the healthcare partnership, but it's a team of healthcare providers that creates the most ideal partnership. Don't exclude support staff members or underestimate their vital role in this partnership.

SILENT PARTNERS: TWO VERY DIFFERENT CASE STUDIES

Support staffers are your silent partners in meeting the needs of patients, but many of them don't realize the impact they have. Some of them don't recognize the value of their role and may not be provided with the information and motivation to be more patient-centered. Too often, they aren't brought into the equation when initiatives are established and aren't given the tools and support to buy into a patient-centered culture.

CASE STUDY

The Ambulatory Surgery Center that Rocks

Christopher Jones, a 50-year-old attorney, is athletic, health conscious, and physically fit, but because of a family history of colon cancer he sought the care of Nicholas Joseph, MD, a gastroenterologist. Dr. Joseph explained the importance of having a colonoscopy based on his family history, but alleviated his need to be concerned. He was warm and communicated well, answering all Christopher's questions. Dr. Joseph then escorted him to the nurse educator, Chloe Morgan, who was unrushed and very accommodating. She provided detailed instructions, obtained signed consents, and scheduled Christopher for a colonoscopy at the Miltown Ambulatory Surgery Center (ASC), which was attached to the local 400-bed hospital near his home. The doctor and nurse both assured him that he would be delighted with the care he received at the ASC.

Like most people, Christopher heard plenty of horror stories about how awful the prep for the procedure would be. And although people told him it was worse than the procedure, it was hard for him to accept this. He feared the unknown, having never been in a hospital or surgery center before.

True to form, the preparation was very unpleasant, and Christopher was quite apprehensive when he and his wife arrived at the ASC the next morning. The admission process was seamless and quick because the ASC had done a preadmission over the phone and e-mailed Christopher with instructions and information on what to expect. They were escorted to the procedural preparation suite and given immediate attention. Christopher was assigned a locker in a dressing room where he placed his clothes after putting on a gown, and then was directed to a bed where a friendly nurse covered him with a warm blanket and communicated clearly on what would be happening and in what order. She continued about her work, hooking up the vitals monitor and recording answers to important questions, before placing an IV line in his arm. She and the other team members assisting her all explained their roles, were personable, and did their best to make him comfortable and keep him informed during the wait.

Once Christopher's preliminary prep processes were completed, Dr. Joseph came by to say hello and inform him they would begin the procedure in 15 to 20 minutes and asked if he had any questions. Christopher's apprehensions were fading with all the attention and care he was getting. Soon the anesthesiologist came by to discuss the anesthesia, the medications being used, and what responses he could expect. Within a few minutes, Christopher was wheeled to the procedure room, and the next thing he knew he was in the recovery room, feeling the comfort of another warm blanket and another delightful nurse speaking with him, asking how he was feeling, and offering him a choice of snacks and something to drink.

Dr. Joseph stopped in to see him, and gave him the good news that everything was normal and instructions about his aftercare, which were also provided in writing by the nurse when he was discharged. Soon he was on his way home. He couldn't believe how smoothly everything went and the wonderful treatment he had received, not just by the physician, but by the entire team.

It was beyond Christopher's imagination that a medical procedure such as this, with the many steps and people involved in the process, could be accomplished with such efficiency and excellent patient service. He wondered if this was an exception and not the norm, for he couldn't recall feeling this important and valued at any other healthcare institution he had visited in the past. The evening of Christopher's procedure, nurse Chloe from Dr. Joseph's office called to see how he was doing. Three weeks later, he received a patient satisfaction survey from Miltown ASC asking about his experience at the center. Of course, he gave it stellar marks.

This is a clear example of how well patient-centered care works when the entire team is committed and shares the same values in making the patients' concerns, health, and comfort the priority. Miltown ASC's care team and Dr. Joseph's practice give patient-centered services that rock! Both organizations have well-trained staff members that are consistent in their performance. They work in a culture where everyone understands the patient is what the business is all about. They recognize that patients are in an unfamiliar setting and have fears about the unknown. They know they have the power to make a difference.

CASE STUDY

A Mishap Waiting to Happen

We would like to share a story about how easy it is to make a costly mistake that a patient will never forget—and will likely convey to others and influence a number of people's healthcare buying habits in the process.

The patient, Tatianna Ashley, had a very disappointing experience recently with her long-standing primary care practice, Mason Primary Care Center, when she sought treatment for a painful, infected spider bite. When she called to request an appointment, the scheduler (an important member of every physician-patient partnership) informed Tatianna that she was no longer a patient of the practice because she hadn't been in for a visit for three years, and therefore *couldn't be seen*. Given Tatianna's age, great genes, and good health, she had not been seen for any medical problem during this time period, and it appeared she was being penalized for this. The scheduler, who seemed very unconcerned and unapologetic, went on to say this was the policy of the independent physician association (IPA) the practice belonged to, and suggested that Tatianna go to urgent care. There was no expression of empathy about the patient's condition or consideration for her long-standing relationship with the practice.

Tatianna felt abandoned when she was told to go somewhere that provided only emergent care rather than to her own physician. It seemed to Tatianna, who was already a bit nervous about the injury and her swelling, red arm, that the practice, *including the physician*, really didn't care about her at all!

Luckily, the urgent care center Mason Primary Care Center recommended was friendly, and the physician was attentive. Tatianna was seen quickly, and her infection was treated. It turned out that her infection was spreading at an alarming rate, and a delay in treatment could have had serious consequences. Tatianna was relieved and thankful, but still she was dismayed that she was made to feel so unimportant by her own physician's practice. She was greatly disappointed by this, and as one might expect, Tatianna has chosen another primary care physician. When she contacted Mason Primary Care Center to ask that her records be transferred, it did so promptly, but no one ever contacted her to ask why she was leaving the practice.

Why in the world did this primary care practice risk losing such a valuable patient —not just her but her entire family—just for lack of a recent wellness visit? Moreover, Tatianna is the *ideal* patient. She is compliant, respectful, and always pays her bills at the time of service.

The possible reason for this mishap might be that the scheduler really didn't understand how the IPA works or that the practice was motivated by the IPA to see patients for annual wellness visits because the reimbursement is greater. Risking the loss of a patient (and compromising her health condition) over a possible extra $50 on a singular visit just doesn't make sense when it means attrition of valuable patients to a practice.

Of course, there's an even more obvious question: How does Tatianna *go more than three years without a reminder* for a wellness visit? Even healthy patients need to be reminded of the importance of preventive care. It turns out that like many female patients, Tatianna sees her gynecologist annually and was not aware of any need to see her primary care physician. But if she had received a reminder to do so, it is likely she would have complied and booked an appointment, and the practice would have helped maintain the patient's health while gaining additional revenue. Instead, the practice lost a loyal patient and the opportunity to grow by treating the patients' teenagers and the family and friends she might otherwise have referred to it. The damage could be even greater if Tatianna was the type of patient to go online and spread the word about how she was treated when she called for an appointment, which could have long-term consequences for this practice. What a costly mistake—one no practice can really afford to make. The big question is, why and how often do mistakes like this occur? Just as importantly, does management or the physician even have a clue that such things are happening, or does the employee have any idea of the consequences of his or her actions? Is this the type of silent problem that could go undetected in your healthcare facility?

Sometimes the physicians and managers of busy practices, particularly those with multiple facilities, can be a little too assumptive about how front-line employees are carrying out their jobs, and have no idea when these employees cause a patient to be lost to the practice because of an avoidable situation. Experienced, efficient, and dedicated front-line and support staffers are critical to a growing, healthy, patient-centric practice.

THE BIG DIFFERENCE

The big difference is quite simple. Miltown ASC and Dr. Joseph have teams that understand and share core values related to how they operate their business and how well they care for the patients. They want to know how the patients *think* they are doing and get important feedback to monitor their performance. They are all about improving the patient experience. Mason Primary Care Center just seems too busy to care. There is a disconnect from the tasks of the job and the very person that is being served. If things don't change, it will be paying the penalty for not being patient-centered. Mason Primary Care Center would benefit by engaging a consultant to evaluate the practice and provide solutions to move the practice forward. This would open the door for healthy growth and increased revenue, but more importantly, happier patients.

EVOLUTION OF THE PATIENT-CENTERED MEDICAL HOME

The joint principles of the Patient-Centered Medical Home (PCMH) were developed in 2007 by a consortium of the American Academy of Family Physicians, American Academy of Pediatrics, American College of Physicians, and the American Osteopathic Association, representing approximately 333,000 physicians. Following is a brief overview of these principles:

1. **Personal physician:** Each patient has an ongoing relationship with a personal physician trained to provide first contact and continuous and comprehensive care.

2. **Physician-directed medical practice:** The personal physician leads a team of individuals at the practice level who collectively take responsibility for the ongoing care of patients.

3. **Whole-person orientation:** The personal physician is responsible for providing for all the patient's health care needs or taking responsibility for appropriately arranging care with other professionals. This includes care for all stages of life, acute care, chronic care, preventive services, and end-of-life care.

4. **Care is coordinated and/or integrated:** This coordination extends across all elements of the complex health system (e.g., subspecialty care, hospitals, home health agencies, nursing homes) and the patient's community. Care is facilitated by registries, information technology, health information exchanges, and other means to ensure that patients get the indicated care where they need and want it in a culturally and linguistically appropriate manner.

5. **Quality and safety:** These are hallmarks of the medical home:
   - Practices advocate for their patients to support the attainment of optimal, patient-centered outcomes that are defined by a care-planning process driven by a compassionate, robust partnership among physicians, patients, and patients' families.
   - Evidence-based medicine and clinical decision-support tools guide decision-making.

- Physicians in the practice accept accountability for continuous quality improvement through voluntary engagement in performance measurement and improvement.
- Physicians actively participate in decision-making, and feedback is sought to ensure patients' expectations are being met.
- Information technology is utilized appropriately to support optimal patient care, performance measurement, patient education, and enhanced communication.
- Practices go through a voluntary recognition process by an appropriate nongovernmental entity to demonstrate that they have the capability to provide patient-centered services consistent with the medical home model.
- Patients and families participate in quality improvement activities at the practice level.

6. **Enhanced access:** Care is available through systems such as open scheduling, expanded hours, and new options for communication.

7. **Payment:** Payment must "appropriately recognize the added value provided to patients who have a patient-centered medical home." This needs to reflect the value of the PCMH's work that falls outside of the face-to-face visit, should support adoption and use of health information technology for quality improvement, and should recognize case mix differences in the patient population being treated within the practice.

To review the requirements involved in meeting these principles in order to become a PCMH, visit www.ncqa.org/Programs/Recognition/PatientCenteredMedicalHomePCMH.aspx.

The PCMH concept moved forward; and at the end of 2009, there were at least 26 pilot projects, which were evaluated for such factors as clinical quality, cost, patient experience/satisfaction, and provider experience/satisfaction.

Between 2008 and 2010, there were a number of developments concerning the medical home. In 2008, The Accreditation Association for Ambulatory Health Care began accrediting medical homes, and the National Committee for Quality Assurance (NCQA) released Physician Practice Connections-Patient Centered Medical Home, a set of standards for the recognition of the physician practices as medical homes. During this period, the American Medical Association expressed support for the Joint Principles of the PCMH. And in 2009, the initial findings of the medical home national demonstration project of the American Academy of Family Physicians were made available. By the end of 2009, political actions emerged with 20 bills in 10 states being introduced to support medical homes.[7]

In 2010, seven key health information technology domains were identified as necessary for the success of the PCMH model:

1. Telehealth;
2. Measurement of quality and efficiency;
3. Care transitions;
4. Personal health records;
5. Registries;
6. Team care; and
7. Clinical decisions support for chronic diseases.

Business intelligence, informatics, and analytics have migrated into the healthcare field and will influence how healthcare is managed in the future.

Healthcare technology is essential for healthcare practitioners to meet "Meaningful Use" standards established through the American Recovery and Reinvestment Act of 2009 (ARRA) and reap the benefit of becoming an NCQA PCMH. The ARRA also resulted in CMS establishing methods to encourage medical practices to adapt to technology in order to accomplish this and be able to effectively improve patient-centered efforts, communication and coordination of care, and improved quality outcomes.

The Patient Protection and Affordable Care Act of 2010 provided even more opportunities to the PCMH. The paradigm shift from practicing medicine as a solo to a collaborative approach is providing a health community for patient-centered care and population health management. The PCMH model is timely and bound to provide effective quality care to patients.

The ARRA incentivizes physicians to implement electronic medical records and meet Meaningful Use standards by increasing payments for physicians that meet these standards. Physicians cannot maximize payments from CMS if they do not participate in meeting these reporting standards, and will actually see their reimbursement reduced. Other insurance plans are developing similar programs and recognize the financial value of the PCMH in reducing healthcare costs, which also pushes physicians to make these essential shifts to improve reimbursement. Recognizing the critical importance of the PCMH, in early 2012 WellPoint and Aetna enhanced reimbursement to primary care providers by between 10% and 15%. Each of these programs plans to grow rapidly. WellPoint intends to make the program available to 100,000 physicians by 2014, while Aetna had planned to increase payments to 55,000 providers that met patient access and care coordination standards by the end of 2012.[8] By August 2011, more than 7600 practitioners at more than 1500 locations across the country achieved NCQA PCMH recognition.[9]

NCQA PATIENT-CENTERED MEDICAL HOME PROGRAM

The NCQA PCMH 2011 Recognition Program is an expansion of its esteemed Physician Practice Connections Recognition Program, an evaluation of practice systems. NCQA declares its PCMH standards are the first and most widely used formal evaluation program from a national quality oversight organization that results in a designation. The NCQA program promotes the goals of improving the patient experience, recognizing clinicians for their efforts, and providing confidence for purchasers that their dollars are spent on quality care. Many payers have implemented bonus or payment systems that recognize the distinction of PCMH recognition and its contribution to improving the quality of care and patient satisfaction. Inevitably, these efforts will control healthcare costs and promote improved population health management.

Revised PCMH Standards

The 2011 standards provide guidance on developing better chronic care management programs, enhancing patient engagement, and improving patient outreach. These updated standards are aligned with the new healthcare IT Meaningful Use criteria. Achieving recognition is based on meeting specific elements included in six standard categories:

1. **Enhance Access and Continuity:** Accommodate patients' needs with access and advice during and after hours, give patients and their families information about their medical home, and provide patients with team-based care.
2. **Identify and Manage Patient Populations:** Collect and use data for population management.
3. **Plan and Manage Care:** Use evidence-based guidelines for preventive, acute, and chronic care management, including medication management.
4. **Provide Self-Care Support and Community Resources:** Assist patients and their families in self-care management with information tools and resources.
5. **Track and Coordinate Care:** Track and coordinate tests, referrals, and transitions of care.

6. **Measure and Improve Performance:** Use performance and patient experience data for continuous quality improvement.

There are tiered levels of recognition within the PCMH program, but practices are required to successfully meet the following *must-pass* elements to achieve recognition at any level:

- Standard 1A: Access during office hours;
- Standard 2D: Using data for population management;
- Standard 3C: Care management;
- Standard 4A: Self-care process;
- Standard 5B: Referral tracking and follow-up; and
- Standard 6C: Implement continuous quality improvement process.

These must-pass standards might be more involved then they seem at first glance and will require some effort to set up in the first place, but they can be accomplished with the involvement of management and support staff, and there is much to be gained. You can start the process by improving access. Just follow our advice and keep the phone lines open—and open the door to opportunity.

Achieving PCMH Recognition

NCQA provides a free copy of the PCMH 2011 Standards and Guidelines, as well as free application materials and eligibility requirements for physicians and medical practices that want to be distinguished by receiving NCQA PCMH Recognition. Simply go to www.ncqa.org/pcmh. Before completing the application process, applicants are encouraged to participate in an audio conference, offered monthly, or in an education workshop, offered quarterly. This will aid candidates in learning more about the survey process and requirements.

NCQA reviews and scores completed applications and survey information. It randomly audits 5% of the practices that submit applications online by conducting onsite reviews and teleconferences and by e-mail.

Recognition in the PCMH program is valid for three years and recognized practices receive:

- A letter and Certificate of Recognition;
- Posting in the NCQA Recognition Directory;
- A media kit that includes NCQA Marketing and Advertising Guidelines; and
- A press release announcement of Recognition to their choice of five publications.

The process of becoming recognized as a PCMH is a blueprint to enhancing how medicine is practiced, improving patient outcomes, understanding the needs of patients, and working with the entire medical community to coordinate care and improve patient compliance and patient satisfaction. Working in the healthcare field suddenly becomes more gratifying.

NCQA RECOGNIZES SPECIALTY PRACTICES

NCQA recently introduced Patient-Centered Specialty Practice (PCSP) recognition. The goal of this evaluation program is in sync with government's efforts to improve quality and coordination of care. Sharing information between the primary care physician and the specialty practice is central to accomplishing this.

Research presented in a recent white paper[10] reveals some interesting findings, as shown in Figure 3.

The white paper revealed that 25% to 50% of referring physicians weren't even aware if the patients had actually seen the specialist they were referred to. It also states that even though primary care physicians report providing a history or reason for the specialist consults almost 70% of the time, the specialist reports receiving this information around 35% of the time. At the same time, specialists say they send consult notes with the advice they gave the patient to the referring physician over 80% of the time, while primary care

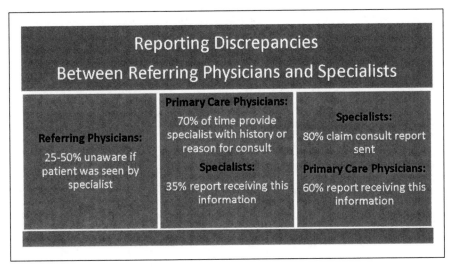

FIGURE 3. Reporting discrepancies.

physicians claim to receive such information just over 60% of the time. This is a clear indication of a breakdown in reporting, communication, and coordination of care.

PCSP program participants are expected to:
1. Develop and maintain referral agreements and care plans with primary care practices;
2. Provide superior access to care, including electronically, when patients need it;
3. Track patients over time and across clinical encounters to ensure that patients' care needs are met; and
4. Provide patient-centered care that includes the patient, and when appropriate the family or caregivers, in planning and setting goals.

The program also evaluates:
- Medication management;
- Test tracking and follow-up; and
- Information flow over care transitions—considering clinical outcomes and the patient experience.

These program elements recognize the need for better care through improving coordination by specialty practices in the outpatient setting, which inevitably leads to a reduction in duplication of procedures and to fewer hospitalizations.

Specialty practices that voluntarily submit results through the recognition program will demonstrate to payers that they are genuinely committed to improving coordination of patient care, outcomes, and the patient experience. To their primary care colleagues, they further express they are eager to be the best partners in caring for their shared patients.

Achieving NCQA Specialty Recognition

For specialty physicians that would like to pursue recognition in this program, NCQA follows the same model used in the PCMH program, by having applicants complete an online survey and submitting documentation of their operational processes and their capabilities to meet NCQA standards. NCQA then completes a detailed review to arrive at a recognition determination, which then lasts for a three-year period.

> *Understanding what it means to be patient-centered is a complex process.*

Specialists who achieve the NCQA PCSP Recognition will demonstrate to government and private health plans, employers, and consumers that they have gone through a rigorous and independent review to assess their capabilities and commitment to excellence and sharing and using information to coordinate care. The recognition can be used as a quality indicator in VBP programs. Some purchasers may make coordination payments available to recognized specialists. In the future, purchasers may decide to expand on the PCMH model to support PCSPs in some way—perhaps through different payments tiers or the opportunity for shared saving.

The NCQA PCSP program is aligned with CMS' electronic health record incentive program's Meaningful Use criteria in recognition of the importance of health information technology to improve coordinating information and clinical care. NCQA uses Stage 1 criteria, available at www.healthit.gov, to evaluate practices through December 2014.

This is a tiered program addressing multiple levels of performance. Level 1 is awarded to a practice that meets the minimum score of 25 points out 100 and all mandatory must-pass standards. Practices that score higher can qualify for higher levels of recognition.

Specialty practices must receive at least a 50% score on specific must-pass elements. Below is a brief description of these key elements:

1. The practice has agreements with other practices to manage referrals effectively, as emphasized in the thinking and experience of the developers of the PCMH Neighborhood and related initiatives.
2. The practice states expectations and monitors its performance against those expectations to ensure a timely and complete response to primary care practitioners.
3. The practice uses team-based care.
4. The practice has a quality improvement program.

This is a new concept for specialists, but their role in coordinating care and bridging the care between PCPs and specialists bring an incredible contribution to the PCMH model and the value patients' gain.

OUR PATIENT-CENTERED FUTURE

PCMH and PCSP programs will continue to expand and be enhanced to encourage more clinicians to understand the opportunities that are available to help them become more patient-centered and enjoy their work more, feel appreciated, and be recognized for their contribution in a more meaningful way. This will change the culture of the medical practice forever. It will improve how staff is trained and increase expectations when it comes to respecting and valuing patients' needs. Patients will know more about their health and be more involved in their care decisions.

Patient-centered programs and the contributions they make will continue to be monitored and measured against the goals. New programs will emerge, and clinician participation in existing programs will continue to grow. How physicians practice medicine and management of healthcare in the United States will continue to advance and will be ever-changing.

> *Many physicians in private practice are not accustomed to being monitored for the patient experience in a meaningful way.*

The focus on being more patient-centric makes sense; everyone wins. Patients like being more engaged in the care process and being in a practice that is more patient-centered and respectful of their needs. They value this type of ongoing relationship with clinicians and their support staff. Many physicians find it more satisfying to work with practice teams that have nurtured the patient relationship and anticipate the needs of the patients. Collaboration enhances the team and results in more satisfaction and pride in what is accomplished. Purchasers, both employers and insurance plans, gain improved care coordination and better clinical outcomes for patients, and they recognize the financial advantage of prevention, early detection and intervention, and better population health management.

Perhaps the most important element necessary to succeed in the movement to be more patient-centered is creating unity across the healthcare system—a culture of shared values and trust among the hospital, executive leaders, and physician community that results in an ideal partnership with patients and a healthier America.

THE PAYOFF

Physicians and medical practices have opportunities to benefit by meeting PQRS core measures and/or attaining PCMH or PCSP recognition. Patient-centered care standards encourage physicians to engage and strengthen relationships with patients, contributing to shared decision-making, better compliance, and improved patient satisfaction that results in greater financial rewards for physicians and improved health for their patients.

References

1. Rickert J. Patient-Centered Care: What It Means and How to Get There. www.healthaffairs.org; blog posted January 24, 2012.

2. Committee on Quality of Health Care in America. *Crossing the Quality Chasm: A New Health System for the 21st Century.* Institute of Medicine. 2001.

3. Epstein RM, Street RL Jr. The values and value of patient-centered care. *Ann Fam Med.* 2011;9:100-103.

4. Harrington R, Coffin J, Chauhan B. Understanding how the Physician Quality Reporting System affects primary care physicians. *J Med Pract Manage.* 2013;28:248-250.

5. Mathews AW. Medical care time warp. *Wall Street Journal.* August 2, 2012.

6. Tibken S. Numbers, numbers and more numbers. *Wall Street Journal.* April 16, 2012.

7. Medical Home. Wikipedia. http:// en.wikipedia.org/wiki/Medical_home.

8. McDaniel D, Dishman E. Patient Centered Medical Home: A Foundation for Delivering Better Care, Better Health, and Better Value. Sage Growth Partners LLC. July 2012; www.sage-growth.com/our-solutions/thought-leadership/whitepapers/ge_health-care_pcmh_whitepaper-2.

9. Allison A. Patient-Centered Medical Home: The Call to Action. Success EHS. August 11, 2011.

10. Patient-Centered Specialty Practice Recognition. National Committee for Quality Assurance. 2013.

Index

Greenbranch Publishing

www.greenbranch.com   (800) 933-3711

The Journal of Medical Practice Management©

Fast Practice: Medical Practice Information at the Speed of Sound Newsletter and Audio

Books and eBooks

Neil Baum/Catherine Maley/Andrew Schneider: *Social Media for the Health Care Profession*

Randy Bauman: *Time to Sell? Guide to Selling a Physician Practice: Value, Options, Alternatives, 2nd Edition*

Joel Blau/Ron Paprocki: *The Prescription for Financial Health: Physician's Guide to Financial Planning*

Judy Capko: *Secrets of The Best-Run Practices, 2nd Edition*

Judy Capko: *Take Back Time: Bringing Time Management to Medicine*

Judy Capko/Cheryl Bisera: *The Patient-Centered Payoff: Driving Practice Growth Through Image, Culture, and Patient Experience*

Frank Cohen/Owen Dahl: *Lean Six Sigma for the Medical Practice*

Owen Dahl: *Think Business! Medical Practice Quality, Efficiency, Profits*

Owen Dahl: *Guide to Medical Practice Disaster Planning*

Jeffrey Gorke: *The Physician's Guide to the Business of Medicine: Dreams & Realities*

John Guiliana/Hal Ornstein: *31½ Essentials for Running Your Medical Practice*

Marc Halley/Halley Consulting Group: *The Medical Practice Start-Up Guide*

(continued, next page)

Wendy Lipton-Dibner: *MAD Leadership for Healthcare: Proven Strategies to Get People to Do What You Want Them to Do*

Betsy Nicoletti: *Auditing Physician Services and E/M Coding*

Betsy Nicoletti: *The Field Guide to Physician Coding, 2nd Edition*

Luis Pareras: *Innovation & Entrepreneurship in the Healthcare Sector: Idea to Funding to Launch*

Kevin Pho/Susan Gay: *Establishing, Managing, and Protecting Your Online Reputation: A Social Media Guide for Physicians and Medical Practices*

Richard Reece: *The Health Reform Maze: A Blueprint for Physician Practices*

Max Reiboldt/Coker Group: *RVUs at Work: Relative Value Units in the Medical Practice, 2nd Edition*

Laura Sachs Hills: *How to Recruit, Motivate & Manage a Winning Staff*

Don Self/Steve Verno: *ERISA: The Medical Practice Guide to the Employee Retirement Income Security Act*

Lawrence Shapiro: *Quality Care, Affordable Care: How Physicians Can Reduce Variation and Decrease the Cost of Health Care*

Ron Sterling: *Keys to EMR/EHR Success, 2nd Edition* Winner! HIMSS Book of the Year Award

Drew Stevens: *Patient Acceleration: Helping Chiropractors Maximize Patient Volume and Revenue*

Alan Whiteman: *Cutting Costs in the Medical Practice, 2nd Edition*